Michael W. Ross
Editor

HIV/AIDS
and Sexuality

Pre-publication
REVIEWS,
COMMENTARIES,
EVALUATIONS . . .

"**T**he chapters presented in this special volume of the *Journal of Psychology & Human Sexuality* address a variety of issues around sexuality in people with HIV, from a multi-national perspective: research from the United States, Europe and the Antipodes is included.

Within the overarching theme of HIV infection, different chapters examine interpersonal relationships, identity changes, quality of life, sexuality, sexual addiction, sexual practices, changing practices, and safer sex, personality characteristics associated with risk behaviours and infection, clinical group psychotherapy, and communication between health-care providers and their clients. The various chapters demonstrate a broad spectrum of research approaches from quantitative statistical design and analysis to qualitative methods to clinical techniques, and which involve cross-sectional and cohort studies. The chapters include research on homosexual men, heterosexual men and women, lesbians and drug users.

The volume is written from an academic, research perspective, yet manages to 'get under the skin' of a wide range of issues of those people living with HIV in an extremely sensitive and empathetic manner. In this way the book should appeal to a wide readership of professional interest, and prove to be informative and insightful for students, university lecturers, and professional practitioners in the fields of medicine, nursing, health care, health education, psychiatry, psychotherapy and clinical practice, psychology and sociology amongst others.

In such a wide-ranging volume, personal bias must influence the reader's choice of chapters which seem most valuable, informative,

well-written and appealing. With that caveat–and whilst grateful for the sections such as those of Schönnesson and Clement, Ehrhardt et al., Adib and Ostrow, and Weinrich et al. which provided a backcloth of statistical information and raised a number of interesting hypotheses for further studies–for me, some of the qualitative investigations were especially effective. Foremost amongst those qualitative works were the chapters by Ross and Ryan, Roth, Schaefer et al. and Cannold et al. They provided an understanding of the ethos of, and atmospherics within, the social situations and psychological processes involved, while being written within firm theoretical frameworks which allowed insightful interpretations to be derived from the data."

Leo B. Hendry, MSc, MEd, PhD, FBPS, CPsychol
Professor of Education
University of Aberdeen
King's College
Aberdeen, Scotland

Harrington Park Press
An Imprint of
The Haworth Press, Inc.

HIV/AIDS and Sexuality

HIV/AIDS and Sexuality

Michael W. Ross, PhD, MPH, MHPEd
Editor

HIV/AIDS and Sexuality, edited by Michael W. Ross, was simultaneously issued by The Haworth Press, Inc., under the same title, as a special issue of *Journal of Psychology & Human Sexuality*, Volume 7, Numbers 1/2, 1995, Eli Coleman, Editor.

Harrington Park Press
An Imprint of
The Haworth Press, Inc.
New York • London

For Badger

ISBN 1-56023-068-1

Published by

Harrington Park Press, 10 Alice Street, Binghamton, NY 13904-1580 USA

Harrington Park Press is an imprint of The Haworth Press, Inc., 10 Alice Street, Binghamton, NY 13904-1580 USA.

HIV/AIDS and Sexuality has also been published as *Journal of Psychology & Human Sexuality*, Volume 7, Numbers 1/2 1995.

The development, preparation, and publication of this work has been undertaken with great care. However, the publisher, employees, editors, and agents of The Haworth Press and all imprints of The Haworth Press, Inc., including The Haworth Medical Press and Pharmaceutical Products Press, are not responsible for any errors contained herein or for consequences that may ensue from use of materials or information contained in this work. Opinions expressed by the author(s) are not necessarily those of The Haworth Press, Inc.

Library of Congress Cataloging-in-Publication Data

HIV/AIDS and sexuality / Michael W. Ross, editor.
     p. cm.
     "Published also as Journal of psychology & human sexuality, vol. 7, nos. 1/2 1995"–T.p. verso.
     Includes bibliographical references and index.
     ISBN 1-56024-730-4 (alk. paper).–ISBN 1-56023-068-1 (alk. paper)
     1. AIDS (Disease)–Social aspects. 2. HIV-positive persons–Sexual behavior. 3. Sex. 4. Sex (Psychology). 5. Health behavior. I. Ross, Michael W., 1952- .
RA644.A25H5752 1995
362.1′969792′0019–dc20   95-21375
                                                                CIP

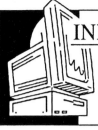

INDEXING & ABSTRACTING

Contributions to this publication are selectively indexed or abstracted in print, electronic, online, or CD-ROM version(s) of the reference tools and information services listed below. This list is current as of the copyright date of this publication. See the end of this section for additional notes.

- **Bibliography of Reproduction,** Reproduction of Research Info Service, 141 Newmarket Road, Cambridge CB5 8HA, England

- **Biology Digest,** Plexus Publishing Company, 143 Old Marlton Pike, Medford, NJ 08055

- **Cambridge Scientific Abstracts,** *Risk Abstracts*, Cambridge Information Group, 7200 Wisconsin Avenue #601, Bethesda, MD 20814

- **Digest of Neurology and Psychiatry,** The Institute of Living, 400 Washington Street, Hartford, CT 06106

- **Family Life Educator "Abstracts Section",** ETR Associates, P.O. Box 1830, Santa Cruz, CA 95061-1830

- **Family Violence & Sexual Assault Bulletin,** Family Violence & Sexual Assault Institute, 1310 Clinic Drive, Tyler, TX 75701

- **Higher Education Abstracts,** Claremont Graduate School, 740 North College Avenue, Claremont, CA 91711

- **Index to Periodical Articles Related to Law,** University of Texas, 727 East 26th Street, Austin, TX 78705

(continued)

- *INTERNET ACCESS (& additional networks) Bulletin Board for Libraries ("BUBL"), coverage of information resources on INTERNET, JANET, and other networks.*
  - JANET X.29: UK.AC.BATH.BUBL or 00006012101300
  - TELNET: BUBL.BATH.AC.UK or 138.38.32.45 login 'bubl'
  - Gopher: BUBL.BATH.AC.UK (138.32.32.45). Port 7070
  - World Wide Web: http: / / www.bubl.bath.ac.uk./BUBL/ home.html
  - NISSWAIS: telnetniss.ac.uk (for the NISS gateway)

  The Andersonian Library, Curran Building, 101 St. James Road, Glasgow G4 ONS, Scotland

- *Inventory of Marriage and Family Literature (online and hard copy),* National Council on Family Relations, 3989 Central Avenue NE, Suite 550, Minneapolis, MN 55421

- *Mental Health Abstracts (online through DIALOG),* IFI/Plenum Data Company, 3202 Kirkwood Highway, Wilmington, DE 19808

- *Periodica Islamica,* Berita Publishing, 22 Jalan Liku, 59100 Kuala Lumpur, Malaysia

- *Psychological Abstracts (PsycINFO),* American Psychological Association, P.O. Box 91600, Washington, DC 20090-1600

- *Referativnyi Zhurnal (Abstracts Journal of the Institute of Scientific Information of the Republic of Russia),* The Institute of Scientific Information, Baltijskaja ul., 14, Moscow A-219, Republic of Russia

- *Social Planning/Policy & Development Abstracts (SOPODA),* Sociological Abstracts, Inc., P.O. Box 22206, San Diego, CA 92192-0206

- *Social Work Abstracts,* National Association of Social Workers, 750 First Street NW, 8th Floor, Washington, DC 20002

- *Sociological Abstracts (SA),* Sociological Abstracts, Inc., P.O. Box 22206, San Diego, CA 92192-0206

- *Studies on Women Abstracts,* Carfax Publishing Company, P.O. Box 25, Abingdon, Oxfordshire OX14 3UE, United Kingdom

(continued)

SPECIAL BIBLIOGRAPHIC NOTES

related to special journal issues (separates)
and indexing/abstracting

❏ indexing/abstracting services in this list will also cover material in any "separate" that is co-published simultaneously with Haworth's special thematic journal issue or DocuSerial. Indexing/abstracting usually covers material at the article/chapter level.

❏ monographic co-editions are intended for either non-subscribers or libraries which intend to purchase a second copy for their circulating collections.

❏ monographic co-editions are reported to all jobbers/wholesalers/approval plans. The source journal is listed as the "series" to assist the prevention of duplicate purchasing in the same manner utilized for books-in-series.

❏ to facilitate user/access services all indexing/abstracting services are encouraged to utilize the co-indexing entry note indicated at the bottom of the first page of each article/chapter/contribution.

❏ this is intended to assist a library user of any reference tool (whether print, electronic, online, or CD-ROM) to locate the monographic version if the library has purchased this version but not a subscription to the source journal.

❏ individual articles/chapters in any Haworth publication are also available through the Haworth Document Delivery Services (HDDS).

ABOUT THE EDITOR

Michael W. Ross, PhD, MPH, MHPEd, is Professor of Public Health in the Center for Health Promotion Research and Development at the University of Texas at Houston. He is the author of more than 200 scientific papers and book chapters and ten books on STDs, HIV, sexuality, drug use, and minorities. Dr. Ross was born and educated in New Zealand and completed his graduate work in Australia, Sweden, and Finland in psychology and in public health and health education. He taught psychiatry at Flinders University Medical School before heading the AIDS Program for the South Australian Health Commission and later serving as Director of the National Center in HIV Social Research Unit at the University of New South Wales.

CONTENTS

Preface

While an enormous amount of attention has been paid to sexual behavior in people who are at risk of HIV infection, considerably less attention has been paid to those already infected. Indeed, the impression one gets is that once people have become infected, those involved in HIV prevention programs are no longer interested. Of course, this is fallacious reasoning–those uninfected and at-risk will be infected by someone who carried HIV, and thus there should be equal emphasis on those who are HIV seropositive. Unfortunately, the comparative lack of attention to those who are HIV infected sends other messages to those living with HIV–that sexual expression is discouraged in those living with HIV.

The articles in this volume address the issues associated with sexuality in people with HIV disease, looking at a range of areas and methods. The opening article by Ross and Ryan deals with the centrality of sexuality to equality of life and identity and the impact of HIV on sexuality in gay-identified men. In another qualitative approach, Nilsson Schönnesson and Clement look at the psychological impact of making changes in the sexual behavior of gay men with HIV infection, and Schaefer, Coleman, and Moore examine the impact in terms of its dynamics over time. Sexual behavior in women has traditionally been de-emphasized also, and as a counterbalance to this neglect are two excellent papers about sexuality in HIV-infected women by Brown and colleagues and Ehrhardt and colleagues, which respectively follow a cohort of women with HIV infection associated with the military and look at risk behaviors in seropositive and seronegative women. Quantitative studies by Adib and Ostrow and Weinrich and colleagues also look at the dynamics of stages of change in safer sexual practices in a cohort of gay men and personality variables associated with risk and infection in both homosexual and heterosexual

[Haworth co-indexing entry note]: "Preface." Ross, Michael W. Co-published simultaneously in *Journal of Psychology & Human Sexuality* (The Haworth Press, Inc.) Vol. 7, No. 1/2, 1995, pp. xiii-xiv; and: *HIV/AIDS and Sexuality* (ed: Michael W. Ross) The Haworth Press, Inc., 1995, pp. xiii-xiv; and: *HIV/AIDS and Sexuality* (ed: Michael W. Ross) Harrington Park Press, an imprint of The Haworth Press, Inc., 1995, pp. xiii-xiv. *[Single or multiple copies of this article are available from The Haworth Document Delivery Service: 1-800-342-9678, 9:00 a.m. - 5:00 p.m. (EST).]*

xiii

men. Issues of intimacy are described by Cannold et al. in HIV seropositive men, both in terms of relationships and their generation by an HIV
diagnosis. At a more clinical level, Fontaine examines the issues surrounding sexual addiction in gay men and its association with HIV risks, while
Roth provides a valuable insight into communications processes that occur, both overt and subtle, between health-care providers and clients about
sexuality and HIV.

The strengths of this volume lie in its diversity. The United States,
Europe, and Australia are represented. The issue includes cross-sectional
and cohort study designs. Qualitative, quantitative, and clinical approaches to the issues also are included. The papers deal with homosexual
men, heterosexual women, heterosexual men, and lesbians, as well as
injecting drug users. This diversity provides a more complete triangulation
of the experiences of people with HIV in terms of sexuality, explicit and
implicit. It is my hope that this volume will both open up the area of
sexuality in people living with HIV and stimulate other researchers to
devote more attention to the issues involved in sexual expression, HIV
transmission risk, and living with HIV infection.

Michael W. Ross, PhD, MPH, MHPEd
University of Texas
Houston

The Little Deaths:
Perceptions of HIV, Sexuality
and Quality of Life in Gay Men

Michael W. Ross, PhD, MPH, MHPEd
Lorna Ryan, MA

> . . . and things like pain, [refers to question on Quality of Life
> questionnaire] "Have you had any bodily pain?" I mean, yes, and I
> really enjoyed it, heh heh! (Respondent 10)

Sexuality is central to the consideration of the role of HIV in quality of
life. Its central role is related to the part played by sexual behaviour in HIV
transmission. This popular discourse on HIV/AIDS attributes blame, and
induces guilt, to sexual behaviour and particularly to homosexual behaviour. The existence of a popular discourse which reaches conclusions
based on premises incorporating guilt and blame, themselves placed
within a discourse which sees sexuality, at least from a Judeo-Christian
perspective, as being sinful and dangerous outside of a strict set of bound-

Dr. Michael W. Ross is affiliated with the Center for Health Promotion Research and Development, School of Public Health, University of Texas at Houston, P.O. Box 20186, Houston, TX 77225, USA. Lorna Ryan is affiliated with the
Department of Sociology, University of Kent, Canterbury, UK. This research was
carried out when both authors were with the National Centre in HIV Social
Research, University of New South Wales, Sydney, Australia.

Correspondence should be addressed to Dr. Ross.

The authors wish to thank Dr. Brett Tindall for his helpful comments and
advice in the course of the study.

[Haworth co-indexing entry note]: "The Little Deaths: Perceptions of HIV, Sexuality and Quality of
Life in Gay Men." Ross, Michael W., and Lorna Ryan. Co-published simultaneously in *Journal of
Psychology & Human Sexuality* (The Haworth Press, Inc.) Vol. 7, No. 1/2, 1995, pp. 1-20; and:
HIV/AIDS and Sexuality (ed: Michael W. Ross) The Haworth Press, Inc., 1995, pp. 1-20; and: *HIV/AIDS
and Sexuality* (ed: Michael W. Ross) Harrington Park Press, an imprint of The Haworth Press, Inc.,
1995, pp. 1-20. *[Single or multiple copies of this article are available from The Haworth Document
Delivery Service: 1-800-342-9678, 9:00 a.m. - 5:00 p.m. (EST).]*

1

aries, has implications for those who adopt subject positions within the dominant icon. In terms of the disease, while the body has been medicalized through a specific sexual act, its reciprocal (the recognition of sexuality in the medicalized) has usually been denied. The major metaphor of AIDS, as Sontag (1989) has noted, is one of punishment for transgressing sexual mores.

This research will concern itself primarily with sexuality and homosexually active and self-identified gay men, since these groups inform the relationships between sexuality, HIV and quality of life. The comparative silence about the issue of sexuality in illness predates the HIV pandemic and may be conceptualized according to the Parsonian notion that illness, and the adoption of a "sick role" requires that the ill person is excluded from certain responsibilities and duties, and hence becomes asexual. However, there is a more general avoidance of addressing illness and sexuality, particularly with regard to persons with mental and physical disabilities and the elderly.

METHOD

We conducted interviews with sixteen gay men who were current or ex-participants in clinical trials of anti-HIV agents carried out by the National Centre in HIV Epidemiology and Clinical Research in Sydney, Australia. We also interviewed six HIV clinical trial nurses, and while these data will form a further research paper, we have used portions of these latter interviews where appropriate. Interviews were carried out in Sydney and Canberra, and some participants were being treated by private physicians, in the community, and in hospitals and ambulatory care centers. While the primary purpose of the interviews, which were recorded and transcribed *verbatim*, was to investigate the experience of being on a clinical trial, we also asked specific questions about sexuality. Respondents were also shown a widely used measure of quality of life, and asked to comment on their conceptions of quality of life in the light of the questions asked. Respondents' critiques of "expertly designed" scales were used as a starting point for discussion of the relationships between sexuality and quality of life in HIV disease, but also highlight the extent to which experts may be unaware of the concerns of people with HIV. Data were analysed by extracting the sections of the interviews dealing with sexuality, and organising them into conceptual categories based on content. Qualitative data analysis consists, according to Spradley (1979), of a search for the parts of a concept, the relationship between those parts, and the relationship of the parts to the whole. We intend to follow this model using theme analysis. A theme is a pattern of thought which connects domains, and something which people within the target area will accept as valid. A domain is considered to be a symbolic category which contains related words. In many cases, the themes of a content area such as burnout and reward may not be explicitly expressed, and hence must be uncovered by the actions and descriptive language and rules of the target group. We followed this definition in this data analysis. The study was approved by the relevant university ethics committee. We emphasise that this is a pilot study and therefore that findings may not be representative of gay men or of other gay satellite cultures, but do represent some of the issues relating to sexuality and quality of life for the gay men interviewed.

CULTURE AND IDENTIFICATION

While Hunt (1966) has noted that the health services, values and expectations of any culture will influence what constitutes quality of life, culture, as Tindall notes, will be defined not only in ethnological terms but particularly with regard to such variables as sexuality, socio-economic status, and employment. Cultural values of what constitutes quality of life will vary widely from group to group and there can be no absolute value of quality of life (although there are key values which can be delineated within a specific and identifiable culture). We argue that where the culture or satellite culture is defined both by members and non-members by sexuality, then sexual expression will play a major part in quality of life definitions, and that sexuality is one of those key values.

Within medical science and clinical trials where quality of life is evaluated, the relative silence about quality of life issues conveys its own message. Where studies of anti-HIV agents have incorporated quality of life measures, in many cases they have been tokenistic and the measures used, with few exceptions, have ignored issues of sexuality. Whether this is due to general discomfort about sexuality or more specific homonegative attitudes ("homophobia") is unclear. This silence itself carries a potent message for those rating questionnaire instruments, when what may be considered one of the more important bases of their identity is ignored. Sexuality, even in the context of clinical trials and measurement of quality of life, has been set aside as an area "not to be named among doctors." This provides a symbolic indication about its acceptability and about its transgression to individuals, who in most cases in homosexual men, may define themselves and their exposure to HIV (despite the political unacceptability of the term "risk group" and attempts to provide circumlocutions), in sexual terms. The silence about sexual expression and sexual functioning may actually serve to emphasise the co-categorization of HIV and homosexuality.

Given that the dominant public discourse of homosexuality is now to a significant extent constructed on the basis of a discourse of HIV/AIDS, our understanding of sexual expression is indexed in a discourse which equates homosexuality as such, and not specific penetrative sexual practices, with HIV. This co-categorization is illustrated by two respondents who indicated that the reminder of how they were infected with HIV reoccurred. Respondent 6 describes how this has affected his sexual functioning completely:

> I associated sex with my predicament, er, something just cracked and of course everybody has different feelings and that, but I mean it just turns me off, just the very thought of having sex.

Even when sexuality continues, the reminder of the source of infection may recur. For example, having to take anti-HIV drugs at regular intervals may be a reminder both to individuals and their partners, as Respondent 15 indicates:

> [about taking Zidovudine every four hours] But at night it was a real pain in the neck especially as, um, if you, how do I put this, if you picked up someone and you wanted to go home that was one of the things about the alarm clock you know, whatever, and back in '88, there wasn't that many people who'd coped with HIV positive people . . . 'cos that was really like how I got it, apart from me being reminded every four hours, *they* were being reminded every four hours. . . .

The issues of identity and behaviour which face the homosexually identified man in the sexual sphere depend on whether he is infected with HIV and the stage of HIV disease. For the healthy or uninfected person, having safe or safer sex will impinge on their sexual activity either in the form of the use of condoms, the avoidance of particular activities, or the anxiety associated with activities known to carry risk. For the sicker person, the need for "companionship" may take precedence with its associations of having someone to care for one. The term "companionship" however, conjures up the image of a substitution for sex, being sexually unfit or old, and beyond sexual interest. For the sicker person, appearance is also an important determinant of sexuality, both in terms of self-esteem and in terms of sexual attractiveness. Some gay men have indicated that they have withdrawn from social and sexual situations because of embarrassment about their appearance. A concentration on bodily appearance through exercise and gym attendance may provide support for the notion of being healthy although infected, but progressive deterioration may cause greater distress if it is from the base of a visibly fit and strong body in which the individual has taken pride and on which they have invested a great deal of work. Finally, in the case of more severe HIV disease, fatigue may make sex more difficult or less enjoyable.

The language of sex and the language of safe/safer sex emphasises the change in the perception of sexuality. The terms previously associated with sex (escape, ecstacy, celebration, liberation, suggestion of release from traditional morality) have given way to those of war (safety, responsibility, protection), medicine (penetration, body fluids) or racial discrimination as in the description of serostatus of partners (concordant or mixed status). Sex has become an activity of great potential danger and of anxiety, and this change from identification to concern will have an effect on security and stability of self-concept. Here, the concept of being discredited, self-doubt or denigration, and for the HIV infected individual the notion of the failed body (Goffman, 1963) may emerge. The result may be self-quarantine, where a choice of being sexual or asexual may be made. This self-quarantine may be generated by the combination of a perception of blame and guilt in the popular HIV/AIDS discourse, fear of rejection and discredited identity as well as, if relevant, concerns about sexual functioning. There may also be a lesser form of self-quarantine which involves a heightened perception of risk of superinfection with another pathogen or viral strain, as observed by Respondents 5 and 11 respectively:

> Yeah, the sex life is important, but I'm not going to jeopardise my health by going out and searching for it and doing the beats and doing the bars or anything, I mean all that, that's past.

> I mean, part of it is whether or not that HIV has scared people off sex–I'm not sure, in some cases it has, um, it's whether going on the [clinical] trial has sort of made people feel more fragile and less likely to engage in sex because there might be the *slightest* risk of further infection.

The messages about the role of sex and sexuality in the attribution of responsibility for the HIV pandemic may also be projected from researchers themselves. Lovejoy et al. (1991) report questionnaire items relating to "self-care" behaviours such as avoiding gay bars and washing after sex, both of which target sexuality and sex as being dangerous and dirty. The confusion about sex may also be generated from a number of perspectives.

If a gay man has sex, he may be seen from the perspective of the popular press as engaging in activities which kill his fellows. If he is asexual, he may be seen by his fellows as rejecting his sexuality or being "homophobic." Any decision regarding sex is fraught with difficulty which may have the effect of making a previously enjoyable and identity-reinforcing activity a source of anxiety, conflict and confusion.

DEGREE OF UNCERTAINTY ABOUT SAFETY OF SEXUAL BEHAVIOR

Even with the introduction of safe/safer sex, there is a degree of uncertainty. Safer sex may carry small but potentially anxiety-generating risks, such as condom failure or the low but present risk of transmission of HIV through oral sex. This uncertainty has lead to the construction of what we have referred to elsewhere as "folk epidemiology" (Lowy & Ross, 1994), in which the uncertainty and conflicting attribution of risk to unprotected oral sex has led gay men to construct their own hierarchies of risk and to base their sexual behavior on these. Unprotected sex between HIV seropositive individuals carries the possibility of transmission of other potentially dangerous pathogens including not only sexually transmissible infections, but more virulent forms of HIV. Respondent 11 states that he only has sex with other HIV positive men, but also comments that being HIV positive has

> . . . made people feel more fragile and less likely to engage in sex because there may be the *slightest* risk of a further infection.

Sex where HIV status is known or assumed to be negative is fraught with mistrust as to the truth of the assertion of negative status, or as to whether the partner is really monogamous. Truly safe sex may involve a radical change for some from their usual sexual repertoire to avoidance of anal sex (even with condoms) or avoidance of oral sex, to forms which are regarded as less satisfying physically or emotionally. For others, it may involve less alteration to their preferred sexual repertoire. These uncertainties will have an impact on quality of life and mean that for most gay men, sex still contains uncertainties and anxieties which continue to be interwoven with issues of HIV transmission.

There may be sexual dysfunctions contingent upon illness itself, the effects of medications, or spectatoring (the disturbance of sexual functioning by excessive concentration upon the sexual act and intrusive concern about sexual performance). Similarly, cruising may be overshadowed by the spectre of infection, and sex reduced to an act associated with death. Development of a conflict-free identity in such circumstances for younger gay men becomes increasingly difficult.

POLITICAL TRUTHS AND PSYCHOLOGICAL TRUTHS

Tensions in attribution of HIV/AIDS may contribute to uncertainty. Such tensions may arise between the popular discourse which sees HIV/AIDS as a "gay disease" which was originally labelled GRID (Gay-related immune deficiency) and the preponderance of homosexual contact as the major source of HIV transmission in many western countries, and between the gay community which has sought to emphasise that it is sexually, rather than homosexually, transmitted. Such tensions arise when the rhetoric is directed at one level to denying that homosexuality is to blame, while at the same time arguing for greater funding for education and services directed toward the gay community because of the high number of infected people. The conflict arises because of a confusion between what Dennis Altman (pers. comm.) calls "political truths" and "psychological truths." It is interesting to note the facility with which cases of HIV of unknown transmission source are attributed to unadmitted homosexual behaviour, and the concern expressed by many infected injecting drug users that they are assumed to be homosexual. Even well-known heterosexual figures who have become infected with HIV have been subject to rumors imputing homosexual behavior. These illustrate the extent of the assumption that homosexuality is the "cause" of HIV transmission as a "psychological truth" by people who would never accept this as a "political truth."

QUALITY OF LIFE ISSUES

The measurement of quality of life has been traditionally based on scales which have been biased toward functioning as measured by the physician or have concentrated on physical function (Wu & Rubin, 1992). While there have been major criticisms of the issues of measurement of quality of life covered elsewhere (Tindall), it is worth noting that in the case of HIV disease the scales appear, with one or two exceptions, to be based on lifestyles and concerns more typical of the heterosexual, married and older cancer patient than the young and sexually active. In such situations, the definition of quality of life is "culturally biassed." Specific attributes of a life*style*, including socializing patterns, sexual contact patterns, and cultural or subcultural patterns, rather than life (such as day to day domestic and occupational functioning) may be identified as being important. Indeed, it may be that the definitions which emerge from qualitative data such as are presented here may be of greater relevance in determining the content and positioning of quality of life. Respondent 10 indicates that:

> My life includes much more than what's on this list [referring to Quality of Life questionnaire].
>
> Interviewer: Like what, spell it out.
>
> Respondent 10: Well, sex, dance parties, doing drugs, um, intellectual stimulation and those kind of things.

Trial nurse 4 (whose partner is HIV seropositive) also comments that the Quality of Life scale used in a trial he is associated with

> . . . doesn't really address anything to do on how it impacts on a person's sort of relations with sort of significant other people in their lives, it doesn't sort of have anything to do with sort of how it has impacted on your sort of sexuality your sort of friendships, all of that sort of thing . . . any of the more complex emotions.

For HIV disease, it could be noted that while such scales exhibit the psychometric properties of acceptable reliability, their validity is often poor. It is thus important to consider a definition of quality of life which is relevant to the populations most affected by HIV and their HIV-related concerns. It is our belief that the issues of quality of life in people with HIV disease are best conceptualised not by function but by Tindall's definition of what is relevant to such a population: the discrepancy between actual and desired level of functioning (both emotional and physical). In addition to the issue of whether there is a discrepancy between desired and actual level of functioning, the *importance* of that particular level of functioning must also be taken into account. We argue that because of the centrality of sex in the definition of both a gay identity, and of its centrality in the construction of HIV disease, sexuality is a central component of quality of life.

> Interviewer: It's sometimes still important to remember that people are sexual beings.

Respondent 12: Oh yeah, yeah, I mean, it's part of life, and even when you're sick it's still part of life.

For Respondent 7, sex life has sufficient centrality in his life to act as a global indicator:

Well, sex, yes, I mean when you mentioned sex I mean, that's my barometer of how I'm feeling is my sex life.

Where sex life is seen as being central to the person's existence (as may be other core concepts such as sporting activities) giving it up may be construed as equivalent to death, as Respondent 15 states:

I mean, if you attack my swimming or my sex or something like that, yeah, I would give up.

On the other hand, after HIV infection, some individuals may define particular aspects of sex as being important; for example, the relationship aspect rather than the sexual activity as such. Respondent 5 reported that sexual relationships were more important than sex life on its own:

Relationships more than sex, relationships, I think that would probably be more important . . .

These responses strongly suggest that sex and sexuality (including sexual relationships) are central to the definition of quality of life in gay men, and must be included in any measurement of quality of life.

THE LITTLE DEATHS

Two major concerns in homosexually active men seem to revolve around the concepts of what we have called, following the apparent domains of concern expressed by our respondents, "Sexual Death" and "Social Death."

Sexual Death. The concept of sexual death is placed firmly within the discourse of sexual identity, and centered upon the notion that sexuality is a core identification for many homosexually active men in western societies. Quality of life, and indeed meaning in life, are maintained by the notion that the individual is a sexual being and that sex plays a part in maintaining identity and self-esteem. Thus, a diminution of sexual functioning may for some diminish quality of life. However, this equation of sexual function with orgasmic sex is problematical, as is noted below in discussion of change in sexuality for the better, where Respondent 10 has a far more diffuse concept of sexuality. How individuals define sex is a central issue, along with how this definition may change over the course of illness associated with HIV infection.

Respondents in our study indicated that sexual issues came to the fore when they were rejected (or anticipated rejection), and when lifestyle changes associated with sexuality (such as changes in venues patronised such as bars, toilets, saunas and discos) were necessary. Specifically, the greater the change that needed to be made in sexual repertoire, the greater the dislocation. Further, there may be interactions between drugs and sexual functioning or between the stage of the disease process and sexual function (due to fatigue or other symptoms). The sexual scripts which can be accessed by HIV seropositive men probably change over the course of the disease, particularly in terms of what can physically be done in the case of more severe disease manifestations. However, the fact of being HIV seropositive alone may, in itself, cause a diminution in quality of life: as one respondent said, "the day I was diagnosed, something cracked." On the other hand, where people are in established relationships, particularly with HIV seroconcordant partners, there appears to be considerably less disruption.

The association between quality of life and homosexuality itself is problematical. The now discredited psychopathological argument that homosexual persons were condemned to a lonely and sad existence (Ross, Paulsen & Stålström, 1988) has provided a subconscious peg on which to hang the notion that homosexuality and quality of life are incompatible: further, as there is the perception that excessive quality of life is the *cause* of the infection through having too much of a sexual "good time." While there is a certain magical element in the idea that self-care involves avoiding sex (cf. Lovejoy et al., 1991), the silence surrounding sexuality in most quality of life measures does tend to reinforce it. Many respondents indicated that sex was seldom viewed from the same perspective following a diagnosis of HIV infection. Change in sex as a result of HIV infection may be in the direction of reduced, or of enhanced, sexuality, but there is usually some change. Respondent 11 said:

> Your priorities change when you get a positive diagnosis, you're looking at the short end of life, you know you're not going to live forever and there's a very real chance that you're looking at the short end of ten years and you make adjustments accordingly and your sex life changes too.

Change in Emphasis of Sexuality for the Worse

Not uncommon was the perception that HIV infection was the equivalent of sexual death, as indicated by Respondent 8:

> So, sexual life, everything–everything just ceased.

Similar sentiments are expressed by Respondent 6:

> Interviewer: Is sex life an important part of quality of life?
>
> Well, it was, oh, undeniably so, but it is not anymore . . . It's just, it's I can't think about it, I couldn't think of anything worse.

A variation on this was expressed by Respondent 9, who indicated that while there was still a generalised sexual interest, he was not interested in being specifically sexual:

> You know I still walk down the street and a cute guy walks past and oh yeah but that's as far as it goes (laughs)–it's better than running down–but actually doing anything about it, though . . .

Change in Emphasis of Sexuality for the Better

On the other hand, there were also a substantial number of respondents who felt that HIV infection had offered them a chance to re-evaluate their approach to sexual matters, such as Respondent 10:

> One thing it's done for me is changed my focus of sexuality from having to involve an erection and penetration to enjoying my entire body even more and more and that's been a change in my life, it's been a change for the good, I, I recognise much more my entire sexuality instead of just my dick.

Similarly, Respondent 15 indicates that as a response to increased tiredness, he began to concentrate more on the quality rather than the quantity of sexual encounters:

> You know, I started to get a lot more tired, um, I felt like shit and my sex drive went down, for want of a better word, not so much my sex life but my, you know, my time was spent in those days beforehand I'd have five people but then now I might have one but have a good hour or two, fucking good!

In this case, the change was forced by an alteration in physical health. It may be that the stage of sexual identity is one important variable in determining whether people adapt or withdraw, along with other coping mechanisms, social supports, self-perception, and a variety of other conditions. As Respondent 10 indicates:

> And it would have had a more disastrous effect, it was only at the end that I started discovering more about my sexuality instead of just sucking, fucking, whatever, but to draw upon my whole body as part of sex. And I think if I was like 18 or 19 it probably could have had a bit of a negative effect on me but since I was a bit older, it's been a positive effect. . . . It's, I enjoy having sex: not, I have to, I mean, I think I still have to, but I enjoy it more.

The indirect function of sexuality may be to provide a basis for feeling attractive and wanted. As people with HIV disease live longer, sex may become more important in maintaining quality of life. This is not to deny the important role of auto-erotic sex in self-concept, particularly to bridge the gaps between fantasy and reality, and sexual release, and questions about sexual *functioning* must not be allowed to get away with the assumption that sex is an interpersonal interaction only, or focussed solely on penetration and orgasm. However, if there is no sex with others, this is tantamount to taking away elements of the person's culture or identity, or at the very least sending it underground. The impact of this will also depend on whether a person considers themself a sexual being whether or not they are actively engaging with others (although this will also be determined by whether lack of sexual engagement is a matter of "choice"). For these reasons, the rôle of sexual culture cannot, for the gay man, be separated from sexual identity or sexual functioning. It is this aspect of quality of life which is referred to in the concept of "social death."

Social Death. The homosexual is also the homosocial. The sexual culture of the homosexual person has co-existed with, and to some degree defined, the identity of the homosexual. Wotherspoon (1991) and Read (1980) both note how the presence of particular meeting places for a stigmatised and criminalised activity produced a culture of the bars and other meeting places. For the homosexual man, quality of life must recognise that a great deal of gay interaction takes place in gay-identified venues or private social circles. Indeed, the distinction between the sexual and the social is often blurred, as Trial Nurse 6 (himself HIV seropositive) has noted. He notes that

... people with HIV, the issues, the things that get affected are their um, their level of energy, their perception of what they look like, um, their perception of their appeal to other people.

Interviewer: Which can be, sexuality.

Sexual or, yeah, it is, I mean

Interviewer: Can you talk about this?

It's very important because I mean if all you get from people is oh dear your skin looks bad today I mean it's not going to make that person feel like they are attractive in the eyes of others–I have a lot of problems with this because I am at that age where I'm not 25 any more and I'm you know getting older so therefore I'm not going to look young and gorgeous any more but that I can cope with looking 35 and having scaly skin and being skinny, I can't cope with, you know, that I think affects my quality of life because I can't go out into the world with a confident attitude I don't stand up straight and when somebody looks sideways at me I think they're looking at my scaly skin instead of looking at me in a sexual way . . . in fact I don't actually look any different from what I did before, it's just my perception of my appeal.

In this situation, the perception of being less attractive sexually will also affect the social–and by withdrawing from the social scene because of concerns about appearance, gay men are also withdrawing from the sexual. The distinctions between the sexual and the social, particularly in a satellite culture in which sexual and the social contact are intricately interwoven, are thus overlapping. It follows that this may also impact on social support, which has been recognised as a major predictor of self-esteem and mental health, and which is often based upon predominantly gay-associated social systems. Social support is thus organised around sexuality.

The concept of family of choice (gay friends) and family of origin may be used here. In some cases, there may be a withdrawal from family of choice (which may be associated with or blamed for HIV and death) to family of origin. The price of this may be a discrepancy between actual and desired functioning and lifestyle, akin to self-quarantine. Reversion to the straighter lifestyle may remove guilt by association, but it also implies regression to a heterosexual model where sex and homosexuality are de-emphasised.

For the person within a well-organised gay community, this may also lead to loss of community support services. On the other hand, there may also be the development of a separate HIV-affected community within the larger gay community, which reflects a sub-stigma even within a homo-sexual culture, a new closet within a closet for some. The removal (by self-quarantine, by geographical removal to family of origin, or by disease progression) of the sexual culture and the community of identification and social support, is referred to as a social death. This occurs when the desire or need of the individual for culturally appropriate social interaction (private or public) is greater than the possibility of maintaining such contact. The concepts of sexual death and social death are difficult to separate but are central to the perception of what constitutes quality of life in homo-sexually active men in our study.

Geographical removal may be one form of social death. Respondent 5 describes the limitations imposed in a rural environment by return to family of origin:

> . . . because I come from [rural state] and I live in a small rural community, ahm, my mother has asked me not to [tell people about his HIV infection]
>
> Interviewer: Yeah.
>
> And I respected that because she's very important to me.

In this case, the isolation is not only from the lack of a gay community, but the isolation of not being able to share the information about his condition, which effectively creates a second closet inside the first one.

Social death is most clearly conceptualised by our respondents in terms of rejection and stigma when their HIV infection becomes known. External reactions appear to be those uppermost in the minds of people when they are infected but well. As Respondent 5 indicates, the community most affected may also be most rejecting:

> And I've had a couple of bad experiences whereby you open up . . . you tell someone, trying to be honest, that you're HIV and the reaction is quite extraordinary, and someone said to me the other day that the most anti-HIV people is in the [gay] community.

This fear is never far from people's minds, as is suggested by Respondents 13 and 5 respectively:

> It's the thing of rejection–that if you actually open yourself up and you're going through a tough time at the moment because you actually want a lover, but you're just not prepared to go out and open yourself up to more hurt . . .
>
> . . . and the fear, that's why when I told B and his reaction was so positive, um, I suppose that was one of the first times in a long time

that I've actually told, I mean I've told them and there was no possibility of intimacy but that was the first time that he continued to make the approaches.

A major form of social death may involve a lack of self-esteem, which in turn limits and prevents the individual both in terms of feeling sexual, and in often avoiding social contexts because they are also sexual ones. Respondent 14 ties this in to the issue of self-esteem in sexuality:

> Interviewer: So what do you miss most, if you had to say what you miss most?
>
> A sexual life, which I don't have because I have no self-confidence . . .
>
> Interviewer: Yeah.
>
> But I've no self-confidence, I can't even go to a bar because I've got these spots [Kaposi's sarcoma] and I have a very small minor case but it's just that. . . .
>
> Interviewer: Yeah.
>
> So basically I have no life.

The issue of self-esteem inevitably also impacts upon sexuality, as Respondent 15 comments:

> How you feel about yourself as a sexual person, how you think other people's perceptions of you have changed 'cos I mean if you're really skinny and whatnot–um, it's not going to do much for your personal feeling about yourself, um, your actual sexual performance.

The issue of social death is tied into sexuality by the fact that many social contexts are also sexual ones, and social and sexual activities are not necessarily delineable, as in the case of Respondent 10, who talked about sex and parties as part of his lifestyle. Similarly, Respondent 15 makes the connection between sexual and social activities:

> And the other thing is, what, cruising and sleazing activities, if you're exhausted you're not going to cruise and sleaze.

The limitation of the social circle by the advanced disease process is also likely to severely limit social interaction, not just in a sexual context, as Respondent 7 notes:

> If you can't go out socially because you've ah got constant diarrhea
> and nausea problems, um, then you can work around it, you can
> invite people over who know you and understand and don't mind if
> you dash off to the toilet every ten minutes.

Concern about relationships also figured large in the concerns of those
respondents who had ongoing partnerships. The concern about sexuality
was centered around the viability of their partner's commitment if sex was
not possible, as described by Respondent 7:

> D can say, I love you, I need you and I really care about you an awful
> lot, um, but a good roll in bed is a lot more to me. Um, also the fact
> of if he doesn't get it from me, where's he going to get it from? If I'm
> a non-sexually functioning being, does this jeopardise the non-
> sexual parts of the relationship, um, if he's filling in gaps with other
> people that I can't supply.

While this paper is about sexuality and not specifically about the social
withdrawal which may be associated with terminal HIV disease, the difficulty of separating out the social and relational from the sexual aspects and
their possible synergism must be noted. In particular, the close linking of
sexual and social interactions in specific gay venues may mean that where
sexuality is problematical to the individual, social venues may also be
avoided because of their dual rôle. However, the converse may not be true:
where social interactions are reduced, it need not necessarily be the case
that sexuality is affected. However, illness may play a major part in reducing both sexual and social performance, and the deterioration of the body
and its functioning is a third area which has an impact on sociosexual
performance.

ILLNESS BEHAVIOUR AND SICK RÔLE: PHYSICAL DEATH

Quality of life is affected, in the person with HIV disease, by the
traditional sick role. This is exemplified by the difference between the
"patient" and the "sick person," and how the person living with HIV is
medicalized upon developing symptoms. However, there is also a major
link between the multiple disease processes and infections typical of HIV
disease and the sick rôle. HIV disease and AIDS comprise a syndrome
rather than a single disease entity, and cover a wide spectrum of illness.
Thus, quality of life cannot be described for HIV disease with any speci-

ficity given the wide range of manifestations and degrees of impact on appearance and physical and psychological functioning. Often, however, it is the inability of the body to respond to the physical approaches of others which causes distress, as Respondent 7 comments:

> I need this physical contact, I need reassurance, I need positive feedback and my body was saying ha ha, you can't get it.

Further, from the point of view of the interaction between sexuality, quality of life and HIV disease, the areas of illness may also provide a connection between the mode of infection (where sexual) and areas associated with sex. Areas commonly compromised in HIV disease include the head (it is a common truism that the major organ associated with sex is between the ears, not the legs) through HIV-associated cognitive impairment or dementia), eyes (associated with perception of appearance) through CMV retinitis, anus (through diarrhoea or herpetic lesions), mouth (through oral hairy leukoplakia or candidiasis), and the body (on which such emphasis is placed in terms of attractiveness) through wasting or Kaposi's sarcoma, as already noted above by Respondent 14. Respondent 15 observes:

> And you get bruising, that can turn people off.

In addition to its indirect effect through altered appearance, the impact of disease directly on sexuality is noted by Respondent 7:

> There are times when, I mean, the neuropathy was really bad, that's basically because I couldn't get an erection.

Thus the most common manifestations of HIV disease have an implicit association with sexuality, and may explicitly limit sexual function. In addition to specific disease processes, the fatigue associated with advanced disease may also limit libido and interest. This was most commented upon, for example by Respondent 8:

> Even if the stuff on sex was on, I still wouldn't have had the energy to even to sort of think about sex . . . if you're not feeling good, it's the last thing you want to do. . . . Probably because I haven't got the energy to carry someone to bed (laughs) and all that stuff, so what's the point?

The appearance of the person with advanced HIV disease or AIDS may also reduce sexual functioning. Appearance, whether self- or other-perceived as poor, will reduce the motivation or desire for sexual activity as already noted and the need for a wheelchair or sticks, or the geographically reducing impact of diarrhoea, will also make sexual attraction and functioning difficult. There may also be iatrogenic limitations on sexuality and quality of life. Multiple drug regimens may not be conducive to sexual functioning, and it must also be recognised that the effect of some drugs may be to alter the ability to function, as Respondent 10 wonders:

> I can't keep an erection for as long as I used to, that could be with getting older or it could be because of taking AZT.

There is a tension between those agents which may reduce sexual functioning (despite the folk wisdom of the effects of a number of common antiretroviral agents on sexual functioning, there is little reported evidence of their effects in this area on which to base a judgement) and sexual functioning. Drugs, because of their promise to reduce the disease trajectory, are seen as "good," while any negative effect they may have on sexual function by way of reduction is by implication also "good" as it reduces the activity associated with infection. On the other hand, where some antidepressants may lead to erectile dysfunction or retarded ejaculation in the male, this may have the effect of exacerbating depression by reducing sexual function. The reduction of ability to perform sexually might be referred to as "bodily death," and while it appears to be a concern as expressed by our respondents, it was inevitably seen as less traumatic than the sexual and the social deaths.

CONCLUSIONS

The issues identified in this presentation are centred upon the argument that sexuality is central to the homosexual satellite culture and thus sexuality is also central to quality of life perception. Sexuality in the gay community has changed in response to HIV/AIDS, and this has also had implications for the effect of sexual desires and behaviour on quality of life. Sex may be a core identity for many homosexually active men, as is illustrated by these quotes from the interview transcripts of Respondents 7 and 15 respectively:

> I think H, the doctor I see in [hospital], I have this feeling sometimes he thinks I over-rate sex, um, but then again, I don't think he fully understands how much sex means to me, I mean, sex isn't a point of orgasm and nothing else, it's a whole self-worth stuff tied in there.

That's very important for most gay men to feel sexual–and to feel maybe not beautiful but you know I can still go fuck, if nothing else happens at least I can do a bit of that.

These comments, which reinforce the centrality of sex to identity, suggest that it may also be possible to conceptualise the impact of HIV infection in terms of "identity death" in extreme situations where the person's identification is strongly vested in sexual performance.

It can be seen that the concepts of "sexual death," "social death," "bodily death," and even possibly "identity death" are central to our discussion of the impact of HIV on quality of life. Sexual death relates to the diminution of sexual function or from self-quarantine, while social death relates to the loss of homosocial contact and interaction on quality of life. A further set of issues which impact on the quality of life of the person with HIV disease is the tension between illness behaviour and the sick rôle and sexual behaviour, a physical deterioration which diminishes sexual ability and which may be likened to a "bodily death." It is clear that quality of life in the homosexual satellite culture is integrally bound up with sexuality, and that measurement of quality of life concerns must encompass sexuality if they are to be an adequate reflection of the impact of HIV disease on the individual.

REFERENCES

Goffman E. *Stigma: Notes on the Management of Spoiled Identity.* Englewood Cliffs: Prentice-Hall, 1963.

Hunt P. (ed.) *Stigma: The Experience of Disability.* London: Chapman, 1966.

Lovejoy NC, Paul S, Freeman E & Christianson B. Potential correlates of self-care and symptom distress in homosexual/bisexual men who are HIV seropositive. *Oncology Nursing Forum 18,* 1175-1185.

Lowy E, Ross MW (1994) "It'll never happen to me": Gay men's folk constructions, beliefs about and perceptions of sexual risk. *AIDS Education and Prevention,* 1994, *6,* 467-482.

McEwen J. The Nottingham Health Profile. In Walker SR & Rosser RM (eds.), *Quality of Life: Assessment and Application.* Lancaster: MTP Press, 1988, 95-111.

Read KE. *Other Voices: The Style of a Male Homosexual Tavern.* Novato: Chandler & Sharp, 1980.

Ross MW, Paulsen JA, & Stålström OW. Homosexuality and mental health: A cross-cultural review. *Journal of Homosexuality,* 1988, *15*(1&2), 131-152.

Spradley JP. *The ethnographic interview.* Fort Worth: Holt, Rinehart & Winston, 1979.

Sontag S. *Illness as Metaphor and AIDS and Its Metaphors.* New York: Anchor, 1989.

Tindall B. Quality of life in HIV/AIDS. Unpublished manuscript.

Wotherspoon G. *City of the Plain: History of a Gay Satellite Culture.* Sydney: Hale & Iremonger.

Wu AW & Rubin HR (1992). Measuring health status and quality of life in HIV and AIDS. *Psychology and Health* 6:251-264.

Calendars on the Wall:
The Influence of Sexuality
on Provider/Client Communication
About HIV/AIDS

Nancy L. Roth, PhD

SUMMARY. This study explores the evidence of social and personal forces in discussions concerning sexuality in client/provider interactions about HIV/AIDS. It unravels the complex ways that such forces influence the interactions, each other, and, in turn, how interactions can influence the forces themselves. The interactions were observed using participant observation techniques, and were analyzed using a framework suggested by Giddens (1979) and augmented by the author. Analysis suggested that such forces as societal norms about sexuality, promiscuity, and monogamy and the guilt associated with their violation influence client/provider interactions about HIV/AIDS. Unraveling the mutual influences of the forces may provide an opportunity to identify possibilities for altering the reproduction of the system. *[Single or multiple copies of this article are available from The Haworth Document Delivery Service: 1-800-342-9678, 9:00 a.m. - 5:00 p.m. (EST).]*

Nancy L. Roth is affiliated with SCILS-Communication, Rutgers University, 4 Huntington Street, New Brunswick, NJ 08903.

The author wishes to acknowledge the guidance of her dissertation advisors, Larry Browning and Sim Sitkin, in completing the research, and the encouragement of Mike Ross to publish this paper.

An earlier version of portions of this paper first appeared in the author's PhD dissertation (University of Texas, 1990).

[Haworth co-indexing entry note]: "Calendars on the Wall: The Influence of Sexuality on Provider/ Client Communication About HIV/AIDS." Roth, Nancy L. Co-published simultaneously in *Journal of Psychology & Human Sexuality* (The Haworth Press, Inc.) Vol. 7, No. 1/2, 1995, pp. 21-39; and: *HIV/AIDS and Sexuality* (ed: Michael W. Ross) The Haworth Press, Inc., 1995, pp. 21-39; and: *HIV/ AIDS and Sexuality* (ed: Michael W. Ross) Harrington Park Press, an imprint of The Haworth Press, Inc., 1995, pp. 21-39. *[Single or multiple copies of this article are available from The Haworth Document Delivery Service: 1-800-342-9678, 9:00 a.m. - 5:00 p.m. (EST).]*

This client had several calendars hanging on the walls of his room. I asked the provider why the client had so many calendars. He said that the client was counting down the days until his death . . .

I have a lover of three years. I 'went out on him' with this guy. His (my lover's) attitude is 'get over this.' I'm scared to have sex with him. Am I overreacting?

Lots of friends have been dying recently. They just give up. I'm not giving up–I'm going to beat the disease. One guy died when his wife disowned him. People in bars look at me as if to say: 'Why are you still alive?'

INTRODUCTION

As the above quotations indicate, the interactions between people with HIV/AIDS and service providers address a wide range of emotionally charged topics. The first is a graphic depiction of a man's final days. The second example touches on promiscuity, sexuality and safer sex. The third client is no longer able to work, lives in a community care facility for people with HIV/AIDS and began his conversation with me by discussing death. The goal of this study was to analyze such interactions to gain a better understanding of how societal views about sexuality influence them and are, in turn, influenced by them.

IDENTIFICATION OF SOCIETAL AND PERSONAL FORCES INFLUENCING INTERACTIONS

Traditional psychological models suggest that human behavior is in-fluenced by psychological factors including repression and denial. Current trends in neurobiology suggest that human behavior may be in part in-fluenced by an individual's neurobiochemical make-up. Traditional socio-logical models suggest that social institutions including political, eco-nomic, social and religious systems affect human behavior.

Following the work of Giddens (1979), I suggest that a number of forces influence human behavior and that they can be described along two dimen-sions: (1) societal or personal and (2) acknowledged or unacknowledged. Acknowledged societal forces include social conventions such as forms of politeness or ceremony that are employed during interactions.

David Lewis' definition is helpful: a convention arises when all parties have a common interest in there being a rule to insure coordination, none has a conflicting interest, and none will deviate lest the desired coordination is lost. (Lewis, 1968; cited in Douglas, 1986, p. 46)

Unacknowledged social forces include "pieties . . . a response that extends through all the texture of our lives but has been concealed from us" (Burke, 1935, p. 75). Pieties tell people how they should respond to an issue even if they have no conscious memory of ever having encountered it before. Unacknowledged societal forces reflect the larger question of the relative influence of individual action versus that of a powerful, authoritative other. In interactions, unacknowledged societal forces may be encountered in language. Humans are constrained as to what they can express (and perhaps think) by what is available to them in the language they use (Burke, 1966; Martin, 1992).

> More important are the grey areas of practical consciousness that exist in the relation between the rationalisation of action and actors' stocks of knowledge; and between the rationalisation of action and the unconscious. The stocks of knowledge, in Schutz's terms, or what I call the *mutual knowledge* employed by actors in the production of social encounters, are not usually known to those actors in an explicitly codified form; the practical character of such knowledge conforms to the Wittgensteinian formulation of knowing a rule. (Giddens, 1979, p. 58)

Such forces include ways of behaving under stress that have been handed down for so many generations that no one remembers their origins and no one does them consciously.

Unacknowledged personal forces are described as psychological. They are traditionally considered to reside in the unconscious, and include such forces as forgotten childhood trauma.

> The giving of reasons in day-to-day activity, which is closely associated with the moral accountability of action, is inevitably caught up in, and expressive of, the demands and the conflicts entailed within social encounter. But the articulation of accounts as reasons is also influenced by unconscious elements of motivation. This involves possibilities of rationalization in the Freudian sense, as the dislocating effects of the unconscious upon conscious processes of rational accounting. (Giddens, 1979, p. 58)[1]

An acknowledged personal force is cognition, the way an individual classifies an issue. Individuals will think about issues differently and these differences will be reflected in their interactions. I suggest that individual experience will influence cognition.

> What the classifications are devised for and what they can and cannot do are different in each case. A classification of classificatory styles would be a good first step towards thinking systematically about distinctive styles of reasoning. (Douglas, 1986, p. 108)

Of course, an individual's experience of any given situation will be influenced by their psychological make-up, the social institutions within which his or her experiences take place, and the social pieties, including language, that influence behavior in often unacknowledged ways. It is for that reason that my model, following Giddens, suggests that these forces not only influence human behavior, but that they are, in turn, influenced by human behavior (including interaction)–and that these forces mutually influence each other. While societal norms, acknowledged or not, may influence how an individual thinks and behaves, the way an individual thinks and behaves also influences society. Because HIV is sexually transmitted, societal conceptions of sexuality may influence interactions about the syndrome and may, in turn, be influenced by such interactions.

SEXUALITY

One example of the multiple influences of sexuality on interactions and the influence of such interactions on the construction of sexuality is found in discussions of "safer sex." Such discussions are influenced by social conventions–"common knowledge" about what activities constitute safer sex. But they may also be influenced by feelings of guilt–the individual may wonder if s/he engaged in an activity that put him/herself at risk of contracting or transmitting the virus. The interactions might be influenced by guilt about having a catastrophic illness–unacknowledged societal forces equate catastrophic illness with divine punishment for wrongdoing. Or the interactions may be influenced by stigmas associated with the sexual behaviors that transmit the virus.

The emotion surrounding discussion of "safer sex" in the gay male community, is just one example of the relationships among these forces that can be observed in interactions. Many members of the gay male community had for fifteen years associated gay liberation with free-wheeling sex (Altman, 1986). Oppressors prohibited same gender sexuality through sodomy statutes and other means, so same gender sex became a symbol of liberation.

Then a disease appeared that seemed to be spread by men having sex with men. Men having sex with men began to be associated not only with liberation, but with death and catastrophic illness. Social pieties associate catastrophic illness with divine punishment. Many conclude that God is punishing men who have sex with men–a position incongruent with gay liberation. How, then, were gay leaders and other concerned people to teach people about the medical dangers of certain sexual practices without evoking the associations between disease, death and divine punishment, not to mention the social stigmas associated with same gender sex?

Part of the problem encountered in decoupling these associations lies with the language we have available for speaking about such issues. There are four realms of social life that language is expected to encompass: (1) natural–less than verbal, realm of motion and position, (2) verbal–words about language, (3) socio-political–justice, rights, obligations and (4) supernatural–god terms (Burke, 1966, pp. 373-374). These realms overlap in social life, and unfortunately, each realm does not have its own terms, but must borrow terms from other realms which fit imperfectly.

In the case of "safer" sex, language from the socio-political realm (public health) is used to discuss issues that are emotionally charged and are tied to perceptions of divine intervention (disease as punishment for wrongdoing). The multiple uses of the same words confounds communicators' abilities to distinguish between the two realms. It therefore becomes difficult to decouple communication about the need for people to engage in less risky sexual practices, a medical, transmission prevention issue,[2] from the unacknowledged pieties that accompany such communication, for example, the stigma associated with same gender sexuality, the association of illness with people who are somehow different, and the association of catastrophic illness with divine punishment. Admonitions to engage in "safer" sex sound ominously like political repression.

The natural order is perceived as being constructed like the political order because the same language is used to discuss both realms. The language used influences perceptions, perceptions influence behavior, and behavior reinforces the sedimentation of language, perception, and behavior. If humans have the capacity to intervene to stop the reproduction of the system, it is through reflection about such relationships (Giddens, 1979). Therefore this study examines interactions and identifies the personal and social forces, acknowledged and not, that mutually influence each other and human behavior, and may, in turn, be influenced by human behavior. I begin to unravel the relationships among them in hopes that in so doing, people might identify opportunities to alter the ceaseless reproduction of the system.

THE STUDY

Interactions between individuals seeking HIV/AIDS-related services and their service providers were observed at two sites: a comprehensive gay/lesbian health services clinic in a large eastern metropolitan area, and an HIV/AIDS-specific clinic in a smaller southwestern city. Twenty-eight interactions from the first site and 7 from the second were observed during the spring and summer of 1990. This paper discusses a subset of the data that is representative of the whole (5 of the 28 total interactions analyzed). All of the interactions cited took place at the eastern site during an evening clinic attended by clients who had taken HIV antibody tests earlier in the week. During this clinic, clients learned the results of their antibody tests from volunteer counselors. The interactions lasted 15-30 minutes.

Detailed fieldnotes were taken during each interaction observed; recording devices were not used to maintain the strictest confidentiality. Service providers were interviewed after each interaction to clarify observations. Each day's observations were discussed with an on-site debriefer (an M.D. with experience in oncology and as medical director of an HIV/AIDS clinic) to obtain an additional perspective on the data, and to cope with the stress associated with observing several emotionally charged interactions.

Both providers and clients who participated in the study verbally indicated consent after being read an informed consent statement. Signatures were not obtained in order to maintain strictest confidentiality. No record exists of the names of the study participants.

Data analysis focused on the accounts clients and providers gave each other of events, situations or other interactions. The accounts actors give of their conduct draw on the same unacknowledged and acknowledged societal and personal forces that are used in the production and reproduction of action (Giddens, 1979, pp. 57-58). Thus, by focusing on accounts, I increased my chances of identifying the forces that influence interaction and are influenced by interaction. I found threads in the interactions that pointed to a variety of influences–in this paper I shall focus on the interweaving of sexuality throughout.

The accounts were coded using categorization techniques described by Glaser and Strauss (1967) and Strauss and Corbin (1990). I first identified a series of topics that might be perceived as personal or societal, acknowledged or unacknowledged. When any of these topics emerged in the text, I marked the text with a code. I then searched the accounts for additional topics and categorized them as well.

RESULTS AND DISCUSSION

Data were analyzed to discover whether or not the data collected conformed to the theoretical expectations. I found evidence in the accounts observed of the personal and societal forces, acknowledged and unacknowledged, described above. Table 1 depicts my categorization of the influences evident in the observed interactions. In this paper, I shall focus on the interweaving of sexuality with societal and personal forces evident in the interactions observed.

ACKNOWLEDGED SOCIETAL FORCES

Acknowledged societal forces include social conventions such as forms of politeness or ceremony that are employed under certain conditions. Sexuality is a key societal issue, particularly the social convention of monogamy which has received a lot of attention as one way to stem the spread of HIV/AIDS (Public Health Service, 1988). Providers and clients in the observed interactions made several references to monogamy and promiscuity.

Promiscuity

In the first example, a client was receiving results from his second HIV test since "exposure" to the virus. He had been tested six months and now 14 months after exposure. Medical research has shown that if an individual has been infected with the HIV virus, 95% will test positive within three months and the remainder within six months. The client explained the situation:

> I have a lover of three years. I 'went out on him' with this guy. His (my lover's) attitude is 'get over this.' I'm scared to have sex with him. Am I overreacting? We only do mutual masturbation . . .

In this case, it seemed the client experienced a great deal of guilt because he had one non-monogamous episode. He was scared that he may have become infected and then might infect his lover. The non-monogamous episode was with a man who was HIV positive which is of concern, though the client's full description of the encounter included only activities that are considered to be very low risk.

TABLE 1. Forces Evident in Interactions

Acknowledged Societal
Discrimination
Finances
Insurance
Religion/God
Sexuality/monogamy/promiscuity
Work

Unacknowledged Societal
Blame
Death
Shame/who knows

Acknowledged Personal
Information gathering

Unacknowledged Personal
Anger/at institutions
Control/of illness/of others/of institutions/of providers/of life
Fear/of abandonment/of abandoning
Guilt

Monogamy

Monogamy has been a generally accepted sexual more in the United States, though not always in the gay male community (see for example Darsey (1981) and Altman (1986)). However, since the transmission routes for HIV/AIDS have been known, monogamy has often been offered as a way to stem the spread of HIV infection (Public Health Service, 1988). The client therefore had two strong societal forces influencing his discourse about "stepping out" on his lover: the general societal prohibition against non-monogamy and the more recent conception of monogamy as a way of stemming the spread of HIV/AIDS.

A second example of the influence of societal sexual mores concerning monogamy occurred in an interaction with a male client who had had sexual contacts with female prostitutes. Prostitutes may be at higher risk of HIV/AIDS than other members of the population because of the high incidence of needle sharing during intravenous drug use among prostitutes and because their large number of sexual contacts increases the chances that they may have had unprotected sex with someone who is infected. In this case the client expressed remorse about having sex with prostitutes and about having what he termed "promiscuous" sex–both violations of social sexual mores. The client explained:

> I'm not having sex at all now. Sex was consuming me. I was lonely and sought company (with prostitutes). Risk of AIDS goes along with sex. I believe sex should only happen in marriage. Now I am in a healthy relationship. We are not having sex. I want to leave promiscuity behind me.

UNACKNOWLEDGED SOCIETAL FORCES

The influence of unacknowledged societal forces was also evident in my data. Unacknowledged societal forces include "practical consciousness," (Giddens, 1979) a force that guides people's responses issues even if they have no conscious memory of ever having encountered it before. Such forces are described at length by Burke (1935) who referred to them as pieties and suggested that they pervade all aspects of social life even though people are unaware of them. A key unacknowledged social force is the association of catastrophic illness with wrongdoing or divine punishment for such acts. As HIV/AIDS is transmitted sexually–and is associated with sexual acts that are considered by many to be "wrong," the observed interactions show evidence of unacknowledged social forces in accounts that associate sexuality with shame and blame (Douglas, 1966; Douglas and Wildavsky, 1982).

Blame

The first example provides a glimpse of evidence of blame. In many cases, this discourse is characterized by long, rambling explanations of how someone may have become infected with HIV. The explanations usually place the blame on others–although they occasionally involve self-blame. In this example, a female client explained that she wanted to be tested because she had been told that a former boyfriend had AIDS. Her test was negative, and the client explained the test result by suggesting that her former boyfriend's new girlfriend had transmitted the infection to him after the client had stopped seeing him. She thus blamed her former boyfriend's illness on his new girlfriend.

> I think she (his new girlfriend) told my girlfriend that he had AIDS because she (his new girlfriend) thought that she (my girlfriend)

liked him. My girlfriend couldn't tell me (that he had AIDS) because she was crying. So my exboyfriend's brother told me. I felt they were plotting. I thought she (the new girlfriend) gave it to him.

Shame/Who Knows

Later in the same interaction, I also identified evidence of shame. I found that in many cases, discourses of shame took the form of "I don't want anyone to know that I have HIV/AIDS or that I am at this clinic." In this example, the client noted that a friend could have accompanied her to the clinic to be tested and to get her results, but that she did not want anyone to know that she was being tested. Again we see evidence of the shame that is associated with HIV/AIDS–if anyone knew she was being tested, they might suspect that she had been doing something wrong for which illness might be a punishment. Whether or not the unacknowledged social forces that I perceive were actually operating in this case, she certainly had something to fear from her neighbors learning about her being sick had she tested positive. A social worker told me a story of another client who had been forced to move twice when his neighbors discovered he had AIDS.

In another interaction a client noted that his neighbor had AIDS. He noted:

Of course I haven't said anything and he hasn't said much.

An implication in this case may be that the disease is too shameful to talk about. If the neighbor had cancer or heart disease the client might mention it, but one does not mention AIDS, perhaps because of its association with wrongdoing and the unacknowledged perception that it is somehow divine punishment. The client's use of the phrase 'of course' signals that he is sensitive to his neighbor's shame and is respecting his privacy.

ACKNOWLEDGED PERSONAL FORCES

I also found evidence of acknowledged personal forces in the observed interactions. Acknowledged personal forces are defined by Giddens (1979) and Douglas (1986) as the forces associated with individual cognition. In this set of interactions, it appears that acknowledged personal forces are concerned with information gathering about sexuality.

Information Gathering

In one case, the client's desire to take the antibody test was, in itself, a form of information gathering. In response to the first question asked of clients in this subset: "Why did you choose to get tested?", this client displayed evidence that she had thought about the relationship between sex and HIV/AIDS.

> Someone I dated had AIDS. I don't know if he contracted the virus before or after I was with him.

She had thought about the situation–a former lover had AIDS–and she thought that she might be infected and have given it to him or that he might have been infected when they were together and have transmitted the virus to her. Because these issues were all unclear, she decided that she needed to get tested.

Additional examples of the influence of personal cognition appeared in instances where clients sought information about sexual practices recommended to reduce risk of spreading the virus. Many clients displayed evidence of having sought out information from books, journals and hotlines. Several mentioned that they found the information to be confusing and in some cases inconsistent. They used this information occasionally to challenge the providers' expertise, but more frequently to obtain an expert opinion about what action they should take.

Client: If we stay monogamous what would you recommend sexually? (He leaned forward placing his hands on his knees.)

Provider: Are you asking me if you are both negative if you should abandon safe sex? No. Don't abandon safe sex.

Client: What is reasonable? I'm embarrassed to talk about sex, but I like anal receptive intercourse [which research has shown to be the most efficient transmission route for the virus]. I've been out of luck for 10 years. Are condoms okay?

The client displayed evidence that he had been thinking about in what kinds of sexual activities he and his partner might engage. It seems that this is an ongoing issue, particularly among men who have sex with men, as HIV/AIDS becomes more widespread. In addition, this client was typical of clients in this setting in that he frankly discussed his sexual practices. That such sexual explicitness is unusual in other settings is evidenced by the client's admission that talking about such things is embarrassing. Other clients apologized for their frankness.

Another client presented evidence that she had been thinking about the safer sex guidance that was provided in the lecture attended by clients while they are waiting their turn to have their blood drawn. Her provider asked if she had any additional questions and she responded:

They said in the lecture to use something with the rubber?

The provider explained the use of Nonoxynol-9 spermicide which had been shown to kill the virus.

A third client offered evidence that he had read a lot about HIV/AIDS and that he was aware of some conflicting medical information. He challenged the provider several times during the interaction. He explained that he had an exposure he was worried about. The provider explained that in 99% of cases antibodies will appear within six months. The client said he had read that it could take nine months. He noted that his exposure was to saliva. The provider explained that chances of transmission via saliva are slim. The client said that he received conflicting information about saliva from two different hotlines.

UNACKNOWLEDGED PERSONAL FORCES

Unacknowledged personal forces include the forces of the unconscious. The field of psychology is replete with theories concerning relationships between aspects of the unconscious and social action. I found that the predominant unacknowledged personal forces were found in accounts of sexuality that involved personal guilt. The importance of guilt is emphasized by Burke (1966) who suggests that when individuals contravene societal mores, they must find a way to redeem their guilt so that order can be restored.

Guilt

In my interviews with the providers who interacted with these clients, several suggested that many people seem to use antibody testing as a way of assuaging feelings of personal guilt for having done something they consider to be "wrong." One provider said that she had had a client who was a prostitute and had a sore throat. The client was convinced that the sore throat was a symptom of AIDS and when her test came back negative, she insisted that she had HIV2–the strain of the HIV virus that is common in Africa, but almost unknown in this country. The provider noted that they are also seeing lots of heterosexuals who are at very low risk. Many of them are kids who are just beginning to experiment with sex and are feeling guilty about losing their virginity or sleeping with multiple partners.

Many of the interactions in this subset confirmed the provider's observation that people are often motivated to be tested out of a sense of guilt. I have previously discussed the cases of the man who had seen prostitutes and the man who had stepped out on his lover. In a third case, a man was feeling abdominal pains and was concerned that he might have a hereditary intestinal ailment. However, he first wanted to rule out the possibility that he might have HIV/AIDS because:

I knew that the AIDS virus can cause symptoms of other illnesses.

He was concerned because 2 1/2 years earlier he had been sexually involved with a woman who used cocaine. He did not know if she used needles, but knew that she had friends who did. Though his concern about HIV seemed a little far fetched, I first thought that it might be attributable to ignorance, fear, or the desire to keep the information confidential so that his insurance company would not find out. However, later in the interaction, he said:

This test may not mean that I don't have the virus. The provider asked if he had had any unprotected sex in the last six months. The client said no. The provider reassured him that therefore the test was an accurate indication that he was not infected. I got the sense that the client was feeling guilty about doing something–perhaps about his earlier affair with the woman who used drugs–that made him feel guilty and that he somehow deserved to be infected. Ross (1988) has also noted that guilt is the most common cause of irrational fears of being infected with HIV.

Control

Unacknowledged personal forces also were evident where control was an issue. It seemed that clients relied on providers as 'experts' who had accurate information–in this subset of interactions–information about safer sex. However, clients also asserted control by challenging the providers' information. Several gave evidence that they had done a great deal of information gathering on their own before asking providers for help. This conflict between giving control to providers and wrenching it back was characterized by one provider as a struggle by clients to assert independence while fearing abandonment. Kübler-Ross (1969) suggests that clients in the initial stages of illness feel isolated from family and friends

who are healthy and are often in denial about their illness. This might lead
to a sense of abandonment. At the same time, such clients often fiercely
assert their independence and ability to care for themselves as a way of
asserting control over their lives even as a catastrophic illness is afflicting
their previously healthy bodies. The interactions reflected that struggle.

MULTIPLE INFLUENCES

In my discussion thus far, for purposes of analytic convenience, I have
discussed the observed interactions as if it were possible to find evidence
of the influence of single forces in each one. However, the theoretical
framework suggests that such forces act upon each other and when forces
interrelate, unanticipated outcomes can occur which can in turn have an
impact upon the original forces. Such cyclical influences are described as
recursive (Giddens, 1979).

To illustrate relationships among the forces, I will analyze one complete
interaction. I have reproduced the interaction here based on my fieldnotes.
This is a close approximation of what was said, but it is not exact.

Provider: Why did you get the HIV test?

Client: I got tested at six months and 14 months after exposure.

Provider: Your results are negative.

Client: Thank God. (He sighs).
             I don't know–but I've read about long latency periods for
             seroconversions and I had contact with a guy who was HIV
             positive.

Provider: There are some problems with the PCR test–contaminants.
             In almost all cases people will have a clear result one way
             or the other after 6 months.

Client: This stress is a killer, I need to stop doing this. (This guy is
             really anxious–tight mouth, whole body tensed)

Provider: That is a common reaction particularly where there is some
             guilt.

Client: I have a lover of 3 years. I went out on him with this guy.
             His (my lover's) attitude is get over this. I'm scared to have
             sex with him. Am I overreacting? We only do mutual mas-
             turbation . . .

Provider:	Has he been tested?
Client:	Before all this he was tested. If we stay monogamous what would you recommend sexually? (He leans forward placing his hands on his knees.)
Provider:	Are you asking me if you are both negative if you should abandon safe sex? No. Don't abandon safe sex.
Client:	What is reasonable? I'm embarrassed to talk about sex, but I like anal receptive–been out of luck for 10 years. Are condoms ok?
Provider:	There is a low risk with anal sex with condom. But there is a 25% failure rate. Two condoms help and we recommend using a spermicide that contains Nonoxynol-9.
Client:	Grumpy out there doesn't even like one condom–Need to hit him with a rubber mallet.
Provider:	What about oral sex?
Client:	What about pre cum–Is the virus as concentrated in pre cum as it is in semen?
	My encounter with the other guy was mutual masturbation but he put his finger up my butt–and he may have had some pre cum on the finger. Does it sound low risk? Time to get off it and get on with my life.
Provider:	Try to concentrate on your relationship.
Client:	Try to get on with life and living.

A key utterance in this interaction is the client's response to the provider's suggestion that perhaps his stress is related to some guilt. The client said:

> I have a lover of 3 years. I 'went out on him' with this guy. His (my lover's) attitude is 'get over this.' I'm scared to have sex with him. Am I overreacting? We only do mutual masturbation . . .

That he had a lover of three years and that he considered sleeping with someone other than his lover to be "stepping out" are indications of the influence of the acknowledged societal convention of monogamy within relationships. It seems that the client felt that in "stepping out" on his lover he had done something wrong–transgressed the societal norm of monogamy. In return for this transgression, it appeared that the client felt that he might be punished–he might have HIV/AIDS. Views of illness as punishment for wrongdoing can be attributed to unacknowledged societal forces that equate illness with divine punishment (Hastings, 1908).

Earlier in the interaction, the client said that he had had a negative antibody test six months after the non-monogamous incident. If a test is negative at six months there is a 99 percent chance that the client is not infected. That the client chose to retest again at 14 months may indicate that in the absence of infection, the client was using antibody testing and its attendant stress as a ritual means of purging the guilt he felt for "stepping out" on his lover (Burke, 1966). Guilt can be attributed to unacknowledged personal forces that may influence people to seek ritualistic means of purging themselves when they transgress societal norms.

In addition to retesting, the client also indicated that he and his lover had abstained from all sexual contact during the fourteen months since the non-monogamous incident. He noted that when he and his lover made love in the past, they exclusively engaged in activities considered to be at very low risk of transmitting the HIV virus. The client noted that he was aware that the activities were of very low risk, but that he abstained none-the-less. Such abstinence might also be seen as a way of punishing himself for his transgression.

As the interaction continued, there was additional support for this interpretation. In his description of the non-monogamous encounter, the client described sexual activities of negligible risk for transmitting the HIV virus. The client had little reason to seek the first antibody test because he had virtually no chance of having been exposed to the virus. The second test was superfluous after the first, and even more so because the client was not at risk–and he was aware of that fact. Thus, the information concerning the sexual activities during the non-monogamous encounter provide additional support for the interpretation that the client was using antibody testing as a ritual means to purge himself of wrongdoing. Where the guilt is too high for purging, irrational fears of infection in the absence of evidence can occur (Ross, 1988).

My interpretation of this interaction suggests that relationships among three forces influenced the client's discourse: Acknowledged social forces–monogamy, unacknowledged social forces–illness as punishment and unacknowledged personal forces–guilt. The acknowledged social convention of monogamy provided a frame for the client to judge his behavior. When he found it wanting, unacknowledged personal forces created a feeling of guilt. In order to expiate his guilt, he first sought a form of "direct" absolution–a visitation of illness. Lacking that, he found ritual means for purging his guilt including antibody testing and sexual abstinence.

A second example that highlights the relationships among the forces that influence the emergence of discourse was found in an interaction with a client who had used prostitutes. He explained:

> I'm not having sex at all now. Sex was consuming me. I was lonely and sought company (with prostitutes). Risk of AIDS goes along with sex. I believe sex should only happen in marriage. Now I am in a healthy relationship. We are not having sex. I want to leave promiscuity behind me.

In this segment, the client directly addressed the acknowledged societal norm that sex should only take place within a marriage. He had been having sex and was not married, and had therefore transgressed the societal norm. Not only was he single and sexually active, but he had had sex with prostitutes, another societally sanctioned activity. He noted that he had been with prostitutes because he was lonely, an acknowledged personal emotion. Loneliness motivated him to transgress societal norms.

But, he explained, there is the possibility of a punishment that is directly associated with the sexual transgression: "Risk of AIDS goes along with sex." His implication was that there is risk of HIV/AIDS associated with sex outside the bonds of marriage–AIDS can be seen as punishment for illicit sex. Such an association is congruent with unacknowledged societal forces that associate illness with punishment for wrongdoing.

This client, too, was not antibody positive. Similar to the previous client, he also found other, more indirect ways to punish himself for his wrongdoing. He was abstaining from sex altogether even though he was in a "healthy" relationship. His judgement of the new relationship as healthy was a cognitive act motivated by acknowledged personal forces which relied on the contrast between this relationship and the socially sanctioned sexual relations with prostitutes. By abstaining from sex even in his healthy relationship, he might purge himself of his former wrongdoings.

This interaction segment, like the previous interaction, provides an illustration of the relationships among three forces that influence discourse to emerge. In this case, two acknowledged societal norms were transgressed: the prohibitions against sex outside of marriage and against sex with prostitutes. The client experienced guilt which is motivated by unacknowledged personal forces. He tried to expiate his guilt by abstaining from all sex. He associated illicit sex with AIDS–a direct punishment for wrongdoing. He somehow hoped that by abstaining from all sex he could stave off the punishment for his previous illicit sex.

CONCLUSION

In conclusion, these examples demonstrate that not only is there evidence of societal and personal forces both acknowledged and unacknowledged (e.g., sexuality, blame, shame, information gathering, control and guilt–see Table 1 for a complete list) in provider/client interactions in HIV/AIDS service organizations, but that there are relationships among these forces. The model suggests that in turn, these interactions can influence the personal and social forces. In many cases their influence is to reproduce already sedimented social and personal norms, as was the case in the interactions analyzed in this paper. Other research suggests that interactions may have influence on societal and personal forces (Roth, In press; Roth & Stephenson, In press). It is my hope that by unraveling the threads of influence evident in client/provider interactions about HIV/AIDS, I might provide others with the materials necessary to weave new interactions.

NOTES

1. I am indebted to Giddens (1979) for the characterization of the major influences as societal and personal, acknowledged and unacknowledged, as well as the notion that unintended outcomes serve as an influence on future actions (p. 56). It is important to note, however, that Giddens was not explicitly discussing communication when he developed this system; he was addressing social life in general. I feel I am justified in adapting his system to look at communication issues for a number of reasons: (1) Giddens acknowledges that language is the medium through which rationalization of action takes place and social conventions are conveyed (p. 40), (2) Burke argues that language is action; all other human action is sheer motion. The ability to use symbols purposively is a uniquely human characteristic (Burke, 1945, pp. 135-137 and 1966, pp. 5-9), (3) Gidden's theory of structuration has been previously used by communication scholars in viewing organizational communication (see, for example: Dow, 1988; Poole, 1985; Ranson, Hinings & Greenwood, 1980).

2. Of course, the medical model, itself, is based on underlying pieties that suggest that illness can be overcome or prevented, that health is more highly valued than sickness, and that prolonging life is of utmost importance. These pieties will not be further unpacked in this paper, but are worthy of further investigation.

REFERENCES

Altman, D. (1986). *AIDS in the mind of America: The social political, and psychological impact of a new epidemic.* Garden City, NY: Anchor Books/Doubleday.
Burke, K. (1966). *Language as symbolic action: Essays on life, literature and method.* Berkeley: University of California Press.

Burke, K. (1961/1970). *The rhetoric of religion: Studies in logology.* Berkeley: University of California Press.

Burke, K. (1945). *A grammar of motives.* Berkeley: University of California Press.

Burke, K. (1935, revised 1954). *Permanence and change: An anatomy of purpose.* Berkeley: University of California Press.

Darsey, J. (1981). From "commies" and "queers" to "gay is good." In J. Chesebro (Ed.). *Gayspeak: Gay male and lesbian communication* (pp. 224-247). New York: Pilgrim Press.

Douglas, M. and Wildavsky A. (1982). *Risk and culture: An essay on the selection of technical and environmental dangers.* Berkeley: University of California Press.

Douglas, M. (1986). *How institutions think.* Syracuse: Syracuse University Press.

Dow, G. K. (1988). Configurational and coactivational views of organizational structure. *Academy of Management Review, 13,* 53-64.

Hastings, J. (1908). *A dictionary of the Bible.* New York: Charles Scribner's Sons.

Kübler-Ross, E. (1969). *On death and dying.* New York: Collier Books/Macmillan Publishing Company.

Martin, B. (1992). *Matrix and Line.* Albany: State University of New York Press.

Poole, M.S. (1985). Communication and organizational climates. In R.D. McPhee and P. Tompkins (Eds.). *Organizational Communication: Traditional Themes and New Directions,* Beverly Hills: Sage.

Public Health Service (1988). Understanding AIDS. Washington, D.C.: United States Department of Health and Human Services.

Ranson, S., Hinings, B. & Greenwood, R. (1980). The structuring of organizational structures. *Administrative Science Quarterly, 25,* 1-17.

Ross, M.W. (1988). AIDS phobias: A report of four cases. *Psychopathology, 21,* 26-30.

Roth, N. and Stephenson, H. (In Press). The structuration of self, disease, and conversation in communication about communicable diseases. In L. K. Fuller and L. McP. Shilling (Eds.). *Communicating about communicable disease.* Amherst, MA: HRD Press.

Roth, N. (In Press). Identity, subjectivity, and agency in conversations about disease. In H. Mokros (Ed.). *Interaction and identity: Information and behavior, Volume 6.* New Brunswick, NJ: Transactions Press.

Sexual Attitudinal Conflict
and Sexual Behavior Changes
Among Homosexual HIV-Positive Men

Lena Nilsson Schönnesson, PhD
Ulrich Clement, PhD

SUMMARY. In a German-Swedish cooperative study the HIV-adaptation process, its psychological sequelae and the psychosexual dilemma of homosexual HIV-positive men were investigated. The focus of this article is to highlight conflict solutions of attitudinal conflict related to sexual behavior changes. The findings indicate that unprotected sex as well as giving up sexual behaviors that are still positively loaded are two examples of conflict solutions. It should also be noted that the conflict is at work even when the individual practices are protected or "safer" sexual behaviors. The results indicate that only referring to sexual behavior data would underestimate the potential of so-called "relapses" to unprotected sexual behaviors. *[Single or multiple copies of this article are available from The Haworth Document Delivery Service: 1-800-342-9678, 9:00 a.m. - 5:00 p.m. (EST).]*

Being diagnosed with an HIV-infection involves among other things that the individual is confronted with psychological, social, and medical

---

Dr. Lena Nilsson Schönnesson is affiliated with the Psychosocial Center for Gay and Bisexual Men, Stockholm City Council, Box 17531, S-11891 Stockholm, Sweden. Dr. Ulrich Clement is affiliated with the Psychosomatic Clinic, University of Heidelberg, Thibautstrasse 2, 69115 Heidelberg, Germany.

[Haworth co-indexing entry note]: "Sexual Attitudinal Conflict and Sexual Behavior Changes Among Homosexual HIV-Positive Men." Schönnesson, Lena Nilsson, and Ulrich Clement. Co-published simultaneously in *Journal of Psychology & Human Sexuality* (The Haworth Press, Inc.) Vol. 7, No. 1/2, 1995, pp. 41-58; and: *HIV/AIDS and Sexuality* (ed: Michael W. Ross) The Haworth Press, Inc., 1995, pp. 41-58; and: *HIV/AIDS and Sexuality* (ed: Michael W. Ross) Harrington Park Press, an imprint of The Haworth Press, Inc., 1995, pp. 41-58. *[Single or multiple copies of this article are available from The Haworth Document Delivery Service: 1-800-342-9678, 9:00 a.m. - 5:00 p.m. (EST).]*

41

threats towards his sexual existence. The sexual scenario is characterized by the expectations of the HIV-positive person to change his sexual risky behaviors into less risky ones and to maintain these changes during the rest of his life in order to minimize transmission of the virus. In addition to this responsibility there are worries related to societal control and potential prosecution. Among Swedish people with HIV there is also a legal threat. The Swedish Communicable Diseases Act requires disclosure of one's HIV-seropositivity as well as condom use when practicing anal, oral, or vaginal intercourse. The individual's sexual existence is also threatened by the HIV-infection itself and its potential impact on sexual desire and/or sexual functioning. The core of the sexual scenario is the sexual dilemma between on the one hand not to transmit the HIV to other persons and on the other hand to remain sexual.

Major sexual behavior changes as to reduced number of sexual partners and increased use of condoms in particular in casual sexual encounters have been observed within the American (Multicenter AIDS Cohort Study, San Francisco Gay Men's Health Study, Vancouver Lymphadenophati Study, New York Community Impact Project) as well as the European (Dannecker, 1990; Pollak, 1990; Bochow, 1988) gay community. Studies also show that men who are involved in a steady relationship are less inclined to change their sexual risky behaviors including using condoms (Tillmann et al., 1990; Connell et al., 1989; Martin, 1987). Many of these studies do not, however, refer particularly to the HIV-status of the respondents.

Data are limited and contradictory with respect to the relationship between knowledge of HIV-status and changes of sexual riskful behaviors. Some studies (Catania et al., 1991; Schechter, 1988; Coates et al., 1987; Fox et al., 1987; Niemeck & Schumann, 1986; Zones et al., 1986) have found that HIV-seropositive men refrain from unprotected anal sex to a larger extent than HIV-negative men or untested people. Joseph et al. (1987) found the opposite, i.e., the HIV-negative gay men more often practiced protected anal sex than did HIV-positive men.

Still other studies have not found any differences between those who are tested and those who are not (Detels et al., 1989; Ginzburg et al., 1989; Doll, 1988; Calabrese et al., 1986). A more diversified picture that may partly explain the contradictory results emerged in studies conducted by McCusker (1988) and van Griensven (1987). Those gay men who were HIV-positive displayed not only greater changes as to number of partners and sexual behaviors than did the HIV-negative ones. They also reported having had more numerous sexual partners and having practiced anal sex more often pre-HIV diagnosis. Subsequently, sexual behavior changes among HIV-positive men became more salient than those of the HIV-negative men.

Within the context of HIV-prevention the importance of attitudes towards changing risky sexual behaviors is often emphasized as a pre-requisite for taking action towards protected sex. However, there are to our knowledge no studies among men who have sex with men examining the relationship between attitudes and sexual behavior changes.

Every person develops a map of sexual behavioral predilections and aversions that may differ from situation to situation, from partner to partner. The characteristics of this map are of importance to the sexual "re-learning" that many HIV-positive men have to do. The individual arena of sexual behavior changes encompasses behaviors that are very much liked (positive loading) and therefore difficult to change or to give up. But there are also behaviors that are disliked or indifferent (negative loading) and consequently easier to change or to give up. It is surprising that almost no scientific attention has been paid to these dimensions of sexuality. However, in the San Francisco AIDS Foundation studies the gay and bisexual respondents were asked to rate among many other variables the enjoyability of a list of sexual behaviors. One made comparisons between ratings at three junctures (1984, 1986, and 1987). In the 1987 study French kissing was the highest rated, followed by mutual masturbation, oral sex, anal intercourse, oral/anal contact, and fisting. The enjoyment of unprotected anal and oral sex as well as oral/anal contact had decreased most dramatically since 1984.

Sexual behavior changes are often pictured as a conscious and rational decision. Dannecker (1990) on the other hand emphasizes anxiety as the motive. Anxiety can, according to Dannecker, contribute to an increased conflict between sexual behavior predilections and practiced sexual behaviors, since the individual wishes more than can be realized. On the other hand, it is possible that the HIV-climate to some gay men has led to a better congruency between predilection and behavior. The sexual liberation movement sometimes forced gay men to have sex in a way that was not always in line with their own wishes and preferences. HIV may under such conditions help the person to justify behavior changes to himself and to the gay community why he gives up certain sexual behaviors (Dannecker, 1990).

When Dannecker's arguments are applied to the life situation of HIV-positive gay men four different theoretical possibilities can be identified as to congruency between sexual behavior psychological loadings and their practice:

1. positive congruency between positive loading of a given sexual behavior and its realization;
2. negative congruency between negative loading of a given sexual behavior and its giving up;

3. discrepancy between positive loading of a given sexual behavior and its giving up; and
4. discrepancy between negative loading of a given sexual behavior and its realization.

The purpose of this descriptive article is to illuminate among a sample of self-identified gay men who are HIV-positive the following questions: (1) What are the attitudes towards changing sexual behaviors? (2) To what extent are sexual behavior changes occurring? (3) Which sexual behaviors are positively and negatively loaded? and (4) To what extent is there a conflict between sexual behavior loadings and practiced sexual behaviors?

METHOD

Subjects

In a German-Swedish cooperative study[1] the HIV-adaptation process, its psychological sequelae and the psychosexual dilemma of HIV-positive men were investigated. The sample consisted of fifty-nine self-identified homosexual men who were diagnosed with HIV and asymptomatic. The respondents were recruited from two sites. Twenty-nine of the participants were recruited through gay volunteer organizations in Stockholm, Sweden. The German subsample consisted of thirty men from the Heidelberg area of whom most were outpatients from two HIV-clinics of the Medical School, University of Heidelberg.

The mean age was 38.8 years (range 18-65 yrs.). Twenty-four percent of the men were notified about their HIV-diagnoses less than one year ago, 26% between one and two years, and 51% more than two years ago (mean: 22.6 months).

The respondents were in-depth interviewed and additionally they completed a set of questionnaires. The relevant questionnaires for the purpose of this article are those measuring attitudes towards sexual behavior changes, actual sexual behavior changes, and sexual behavior loadings.

Assessment

Attitudes towards sexual behavior changes. We developed a 16-item-scale measuring perceived degree of difficulties related to sexual behavioral changes ranging from "great difficulties" to "positive reinterpretation of difficulties."

Every item was answered either "yes," "no" or "partly." Examples of items: "It is necessary to change my sex life but it is not easy"; "I go on as before"; "It is no problem for me to give up certain sexual behaviors."

Sexual behavior changes after the HIV-diagnoses were assessed by means of 15 sexual behaviors. In addition the Swedish sample responded to another six behaviors covering protected oral sex and protected anal sex with/without ejaculation. The categories of each behavior were: "have never practiced it," "don't practice it any more," "rarely practice it today," "continue to practice it as before," and "practice it more often now."

In order to assess sexual behavior loadings a questionnaire was designed including 12 different sexual behaviors (Clement, 1992). In the Swedish sample the participants were asked to respond to additionally 10 behaviors (oral and anal sex with condoms, with/without ejaculation as well as active and passive rimming). The respondent was asked to mark degree of associated difficulties in giving up each of the 12/22 behaviors. The categories were: "I can't give it up"; "It is difficult for me to give it up"; "I can easily give it up"; and "I don't like to practice it."

A given sexual behavior was assessed as being of a positive loading when categories of "I can't give it up" or "It is difficult for me to give it up" were marked. A sexual behavior was assessed as negatively loaded when "I can easily give it up" and "I don't like to practice it" were marked.

Congruency/incongruency between sexual behavior loadings and practiced sexual behaviors was measured by means of combining data as to sexual behavior of today and sexual behavior loadings.

RESULTS

Attitudes Towards Sexual Behavior Changes

The vast majority of the men (93%) acknowledged the sadness of their sexual limitations (Table 1). This item followed by another five items all assented to items that explicitly or implicitly pointed to the necessity to change risky sexual behaviors despite its related difficulties. However, 79% of the men agreed that they were not always successful in restricting their sexual behaviors. Almost half of the sample (49%) partly acknowledged that they could not change or give up their sexual life.

A minority–at the most only one fourth–of the respondents affirmed to items that reflected more of an egoistic attitude or indecision as to chang-

TABLE 1. Distribution Frequency of Attitudes Towards Sexual Behavior Changes (N = 59)

I often find it so sad with these restrictions	Yes	42%
	Partly	51%
	No	7%
First of all I've to be concerned about my partner	Yes	46%
	Partly	46%
	No	8%
It's necessary to change my sex life, but it is not easy	Yes	49%
	Partly	41%
	No	10%
As a result of my HIV-infection, I've become so aware about my sex life	Yes	29%
	Partly	54%
	No	17%
I'm not always successful in restricting my sex life	Yes	9%
	Partly	70%
	No	21%
I take it for granted to restrict my sex life	Yes	31%
	Partly	42%
	No	27%
I've always been responsible when it comes to sex	Yes	15%
	Partly	54%
	No	31%
I can't change my sex life, it's a part of me that I can't give up	Yes	7%
	Partly	49%
	No	44%
To give up is no problem	Yes	7%
	Partly	34%
	No	59%
I've not made up my mind yet	Yes	2%
	Partly	22%
	No	76%

I experience my sexuality as more intense after I've made sexual behavior changes	Yes	5%
	Partly	17%
	No	78%
I go on as before	Yes	2%
	Partly	15%
	No	83%
I'm completely indifferent whether I expose myself to additional risks or not	Yes	0%
	Partly	14%
	No	86%
Generally speaking, my sex life has been enriched through the HIV-infection	Yes	3%
	Partly	9%
	No	88%
So far I've not thought of changing my sex life	Yes	0%
	Partly	10%
	No	90%
Since I'm already infected it's quite indifferent to me whether I infect another person	Yes	0%
	Partly	5%
	No	95%

ing sexual behavioral patterns. Only one of the participants reported that he could not make a decision. The same holds for "Since I am already infected I don't care if I infect someone else."

Between 12%-22% of the participants acknowledged to the more positive oriented items or an unproblematic attitude towards changes. Forty-one percent declared that there was no problem to them to change.

In summary it could be said that among the HIV-positive gay men there was an awareness of the associated difficulties to sexual behavior changes but at the same time the changes were recommended and emphasized. Egoistic/careless and indecisive attitudes as well as more positive loaded attitudes were only partly approved of and by the most by one fourth of the men.

Sexual Behavior Changes

The results are shown in Table 2. It becomes very clear that major sexual behavior changes have occurred within the German-Swedish sample. Mutual masturbation was more often practiced than before HIV-diagnosis. About three quarters of the respondents had in casual sexual en-

TABLE 2. Changes in Sexual Behaviors Since the HIV-Diagnosis

	Steady partner	Casual sexual partner
Mutual Masturbation		
Have never practiced it	0%	2%
Don't practice it anymore	4%	2%
Rarely practice it	19%	23%
Cont. to practice it as before	23%	33%
Practice it more often now	54%	40%
	(N = 26)	(N = 43)
Receptive Oral-Genital Sex with Ejaculation		
Have never practiced it	27%	10%
Don't practice it anymore	35%	63%
Rarely practice it	23%	20%
Cont. to practice it as before	15%	8%
Practice it more often now	0%	0%
	(N = 26)	(N = 40)
Receptive Oral-Genital Sex without Ejaculation		
Have never practiced it	15%	5%
Don't practice it anymore	19%	26%
Rarely practice it	39%	31%
Cont. to practice it as before	23%	38%
Practice it more often now	4%	0%
	(N = 26)	(N = 42)
Insertive Oral-Genital Sex with Ejaculation		
Have never practiced it	16%	8%
Don't practice it anymore	68%	75%
Rarely practice it	0%	10%
Cont. to practice it as before	16%	8%
Practice it more often now	0%	0%
	(N = 25)	(N = 40)
Insertive Oral-Genital Sex without Ejaculation		
Have never practiced it	12%	2%
Don't practice it anymore	40%	31%
Rarely practice it	20%	33%
Cont. to practice it as before	28%	33%
Practice it more often now	0%	0%
	(N = 25)	(N = 42)

	Steady partner	Casual sexual partner
Receptive Anal Sex without Condom with Ejaculation		
Have never practiced it	16%	8%
Don't practice it anymore	68%	74%
Rarely practice it	12%	13%
Cont. to practice it as before	4%	5%
Practice it more often now	0%	0%
	(N = 25)	(N = 39)
Receptive Anal Sex without Condom without Ejaculation		
Have never practiced it	20%	8%
Don't practice it anymore	52%	58%
Rarely practice it	12%	23%
Cont. to practice it as before	16%	13%
Practice it more often now	0%	0%
	(N = 25)	(N = 40)
Insertive Anal Sex without Condom with Ejaculation		
Have never practiced it	32%	20%
Don't practice it anymore	64%	70%
Rarely practice it	0%	3%
Cont. to practice it as before	4%	8%
Practice it more often now	0%	0%
	(N = 25)	(N = 40)
Insertive Anal Sex without Condom without Ejaculation		
Have never practiced it	36%	15%
Don't practice it anymore	48%	60%
Rarely practice it	0%	13%
Cont. to practice it as before	16%	13%
Practice it more often now	0%	0%
	(N = 24)	(N = 41)
Receptive Anal Sex with Condom		
Have never practiced it	21%	7%
Don't practice it anymore	17%	12%
Rarely practice it	25%	32%
Cont. to practice it as before	25%	32%
Practice it more often now	12%	17%
	(N = 24)	(N = 41)

TABLE 2 (continued)

	Steady partner	Casual sexual partner
Insertive Anal Sex with Condom		
Have never practiced it	33%	12%
Don't practice it anymore	17%	10%
Rarely practice it	17%	29%
Cont. to practice it as before	21%	37%
Practice it more often now	12%	12%
	(N = 24)	(N = 41)
Receptive Rimming		
Have never practiced it	29%	12%
Don't practice it anymore	50%	60%
Rarely practice it	8%	19%
Cont. to practice it as before	13%	7%
Practice it more often now	0%	2%
	(N = 24)	(N = 42)
Active Rimming		
Have never practiced it	39%	21%
Don't practice it anymore	35%	48%
Rarely practice it	4%	14%
Cont. to practice it as before	22%	14%
Practice it more often now	0%	2%
	(N = 23)	(N = 42)
Receptive Fisting		
Have never practiced it	83%	71%
Don't practice it anymore	13%	19%
Rarely practice it	0%	5%
Cont. to practice it as before	4%	2%
Practice it more often now	0%	2%
	(N = 23)	(N = 42)
Insertive Fisting		
Have never practiced it	74%	67%
Don't practice it anymore	17%	21%
Rarely practice it	0%	2%
Cont. to practice it as before	9%	7%
Practice it more often now	0%	2%
	(N = 23)	(N = 42)

counters given up unprotected oral and anal intercourse with ejaculation. Those men who continued to practice these behaviors had reduced their frequencies.

The vast majority of the men (78-81%) used condoms when practicing anal sex with casual partners. The equivalent figures with a steady partner were 50-62%. A small group of 7-12% reported that they had never had protected anal sex with casual partners and the equivalent figures for regular partners were 21-33%. The most clear trend in these data is the giving up of unprotected oral and anal intercourse, whereas there was an increase in mutual masturbation (40-54%). Condom use when practicing anal sex was quite high, but it is noteworthy that 10-17% of the participants had given up protected anal sex after the diagnosis. Just as noteworthy is that about 19-23% of the men had reduced mutual masturbation.

Within the Swedish sample it was a trend to make use of double protection (condom use and no ejaculation) when practicing active anal sex (58%) and passive oral sex (63%).

Among the 59 respondents, 15 of them reported that they had had unprotected oral and/or anal sex to ejaculation with a casual partner at least once after notification of their HIV-diagnosis.

Sexual Behavior Loadings

Table 3 indicates that masturbation was the highest positively rated sexual behavior (88%) followed by mutual masturbation (65%). The active role in unprotected anal and oral intercourse without ejaculation was positively loaded (56% and 56% respectively). These data indicate that the positive loadings of anal and oral sex appeared to be more associated with penetration than ejaculation. This finding was more salient for oral sex (difference between positive loading of oral sex with versus without ejaculation: 35% receptive and 26% insertive) than for anal sex (difference: 14% receptive and 18% insertive). Only two of the participants rated insertive and receptive fisting as positive whereas 76% reported negative loadings. A minority disliked ejaculation from the partner in receptive oral sex (28%), receptive anal sex (20-24%) and insertive anal sex (12-24%).

Among the Swedish gay men the majority reported active protected anal sex to be positively loaded (without ejaculation: 83%; with ejaculation: 63%). In contrast, passive protected anal sex had a negative loading, and so had passive and active protected oral sex (in particular with ejaculation, 79% and 83% respectively).

TABLE 3. Positive and Negative Sexual Behavior Loadings (47 < = N < = 50)

Masturbation
I can't give it up	72%
It is difficult for me to give it up	16%
I can easily give it up	8%
I don't like to practice it	4%

Mutual Masturbation
I can't give it up	38%
It is difficult for me to give it up	27%
I can easily give it up	31%
I don't like to practice it	4%

Receptive Oral Genital Sex with Ejaculation
I can't give it up	0%
It is difficult for me to give it up	21%
I can easily give it up	51%
I don't like to practice it	28%

Receptive Oral Genital Sex without Ejaculation
I can't give it up	8%
It is difficult for me to give it up	48%
I can easily give it up	37%
I don't like to practice it	6%

Insertive Oral Genital Sex with Ejaculation
I can't give it up	2%
It is difficult for me to give it up	22%
I can easily give it up	55%
I don't like to practice it	20%

Insertive Oral Genital Sex without Ejaculation
I can't give it up	6%
It is difficult for me to give it up	44%
I can easily give it up	44%
I don't like to practice it	6%

Receptive Anal Sex without Condom with Ejaculation
I can't give it up	6%
It is difficult for me to give it up	22%
I can easily give it up	48%
I don't like to practice it	24%

Receptive Anal Sex without Condom without Ejaculation
I can't give it up	12%
It is difficult for me to give it up	30%
I can easily give it up	38%
I don't like to practice it	20%

Insertive Anal Sex without Condom with Ejaculation
I can't give it up	6%
It is difficult for me to give it up	32%
I can easily give it up	38%
I don't like to practice it	24%

Insertive Anal Sex without Condom without Ejaculation
I can't give it up	12%
It is difficult for me to give it up	44%
I can easily give it up	31%
I don't like to practice it	12%

Receptive Fisting
I can't give it up	0%
It is difficult for me to give it up	4%
I can easily give it up	20%
I don't like to practice it	76%

Insertive Fisting
I can't give it up	0%
It is difficult for me to give it up	4%
I can easily give it up	20%
I don't like to practice it	76%

Congruency/Incongruency Between Sexual Behavior Loadings and Practiced Sexual Behaviors

Table 4 shows the congruence/incongruency between sexual behavior psychological loadings and practiced sexual behavior. Masturbation and mutual masturbation were practiced in concordance with a positive, or at least a neutral, loading.[2]

There was less congruency between loadings and practices when it came to oral and anal sex; a larger group of respondents had given up positively loaded sexual behaviors ranging from 8% (receptive unprotected anal sex) to 34% (insertive unprotected oral sex). It was much less common to go on practicing behaviors that were negatively loaded (anal sex 8% and oral sex 2%).

Over fifty percent of the Swedish sample practiced protected passive anal sex despite its negative loading.

DISCUSSION

The data presented in this article display two patterns of sexual behavior among a German-Swedish sample of HIV-positive gay men. The large

TABLE 4. Congruency Between Sexual Behavior Loadings and Sexual Behaviors (N = 48)

Masturbation	
Positive congruency	98%
Negative congruency	2%
Positive loading/giving up	0%
Negative loading/practiced	0%
Mutual Masturbation	
Positive congruency	94%
Negative congruency	2%
Positive loading/giving up	2%
Negative loading/practiced	2%
Insertive Oral Genital Sex	
Positive congruency	62%
Negative congruency	2%
Positive loading/giving up	34%
Negative loading/practiced	2%
Receptive Oral Genital Sex	
Positive congruency	74%
Negative congruency	7%
Positive loading/giving up	20%
Negative loading/practiced	0%
Insertive Anal Sex	
Positive congruency	71%
Negative congruency	4%
Positive loading/giving up	17%
Negative loading/practiced	8%
Receptive Anal Sex	
Positive congruency	75%
Negative congruency	8%
Positive loading/giving up	8%
Negative loading/practiced	8%

majority avoid infecting others by using condoms or by giving up oral and/or anal sex. An important change is the shift from oral and anal sex to masturbation. On the other hand, risks of HIV-transmission are not totally excluded. A minority of the respondents (N = 15) still practice unprotected sexual behaviors (see Clement, 1992 for a detailed analysis). These sexual behavior patterns are both accompanied by attitudes that support the necessity to change risky sexual behaviors and those that formulate difficulties in doing so.

The findings are interpreted in terms of an attitudinal conflict as to sexual behavior changes that can be solved in different ways. Unprotected sex as well as giving up sexual behaviors that are still positively loaded are two examples of conflict solutions. It should also be noted that the conflict is at work even when the individual practices protected or "safer" sexual behaviors. The results indicate that only referring to sexual behavior data would underestimate the potential of so-called "relapses" to unprotected sexual behaviors.

The sexual dilemma of HIV-positive gay men is very often looked upon from solely a cognitive and rational perspective. But in order to give justice to its complexity, psychological aspects of sexualities have to be addressed. The dilemma may cause frustration and stress as the hedonistic dimension of sexuality is reduced. The psychological pain is, however, not only related to behavioral changes and/or behavioral giving up but also to the regressive dimension of sexuality; i.e., to give in physically and psychologically to another person. The HIV-positive person is, due to the infectiousness of HIV, partly debarred from this dimension.

Another potential contributing factor to the pain is the psychological representation of a given sexual behavior. If unprotected anal intercourse, for example, represents a merger with one's partner it is the behavior as such in combination with this symbol that the HIV-positive person has to give up. The psychic equilibrium of the HIV-positive person is very much threatened by various HIV-related strains and stressors. The individual sexuality plays an important role as a compensation strategy of the more or less instable equilibrium. Schorsch (1989) has identified three aspects of sexualities: the narcissistic, the relational, and the psychological reproductive aspects.

The narcissistic aspect refers to the role of sex as a psychic stabilizer (or a distracting mechanism) by for example soothing depression and anxiety, reducing tension, increasing (but also masking) low self-esteem.

The relational aspect. The HIV-positive person's sexual life can be less frustrating when his partner is HIV-positive as well rather than HIV-negative or untested. But the intimacy sphere can be troublesome related to worries about who will be the first to develop HIV-related symptoms/diseases and/or die, etc. The HIV-positive person can also experience worries about being abandoned regardless of the partner's status. Single men may worry about not finding a partner.

The psychological reproductive aspect alludes to irrational fantasies about "life reproduction." Sexuality is here viewed as the counterweight for death. Subsequently sex gets an existential value, symbolizing participation in life and its continuity. The need to be sexual and to act upon it is associated with a hope of future and a longing for not being extinguished.

The narcissistic, the relational and the psychological reproductive aspects may in other words serve as a protective shield (or a distracting, defensive mechanism) towards strains and distress. The sexual encounter can, provided the individual experiences feelings of being attractive, affirmed, liked, or loved, become a counterbalance to feared or real devaluation of himself and alienation.

The sexual dilemma may be "solved" in different ways. One solution is to go on living in sexual abstinence. Another solution is to try to find one's partner(s) within the Body Positive group. The individual may also develop sexual depression in terms of reduced sexual desire and/or erectile dysfunctions as a response to anxiety of infecting another person. In future research it is of greatest importance to pay attention to these above mentioned psychological aspects of sexualities, including sexual behavior psychological loadings, in order to broaden and deepen our understanding of the sexual dilemma. Another important research issue is to examine the ways in which HIV-positive people psychologically try to deal with the conflict of giving up sexual behaviors that are positively loaded in particular.

Whereas HIV-related psycho-sexuo-social research has mainly focused on sexual risk-reduction and its contributing factors, our empirical knowledge is almost non-existent with respect to what extent HIV-positive gay men may experience psychological and/or sexual distress as a consequence of their sexual behavior changes. Clinical experiences indicate for example that sexual risk reduction distress may be reinforced for those men who, prior to the HIV-diagnosis, to a large extent made use of their sexuality as a defense mechanism towards mental suffering. It is suggested that whether sexual risk reduction distress ultimately manifest itself in various psychological and/or sexual symptoms is dependent upon intervening psychological mechanisms. Examples of such mechanisms or buffers are personality dimensions, coping styles, coping strategies and attitudes towards sexual behavior changes.

Finally, both scientists and clinicians are in an urgent need to develop theoretical models in order to illuminate the complex web of psycho-dynamic, cognitive, and social aspects of the sexual dilemma of HIV-positive persons. These models could serve as guidelines for future research and to the clinicians as instruments in facilitating individual endeavour to achieve a psychic equilibrium between HIV-infection, sexual dilemma, and sexual well-being. By promoting sexual well-being, we will also contribute to prevention of HIV transmission.

NOTES

1. Principal investigator of the Swedish project was Lena Nilsson Schönnesson and the project was financially supported by the Swedish Council for Social Research, the Swedish Medical Research Council, and the Swedish Red Cross. Principal investigator of the German project was Ulrich Clement and the project was financially supported by the Ministry of Science and Art, Baden-Wuerttemberg.

2. It should be noted that "positive congruency" of oral and oral sex includes unprotected, protected, with and without ejaculation. The focus is which *behavior* as such is preferred and also practiced.

REFERENCES

Bochow, M. (1988). Wie leben schwule Männer heute? Bericht uber eine Befragung im Auftrag der Deutschen AIDS-Hilfe. Berlin: AIDS-Forum D.A:H., Band II.

Calabrese, L.H., Buck, H., Easley, K.A., & Proffitt, M.R. (1986). Persistence of high risk sexual activity among homosexual men in an area of low incidence for acquired immunodeficiency syndrome. AIDS Research 2:357-361.

Catania, J.A., Coates, T. J., Stall, R., Bye, L., Kegeles, S.M. m fl. (1991). Changes in condom use among homosexual men in San Francisco. Health Psychology, 10(3):190-199.

Clement, U. (1992). HIV-positiv. Psychische Verarbeitung, subjektive Infektionstheorien und psychosexuelle Konflikte HIV-Infizierter. Eine komparativ-kasuistische Studie. Stuttgart: Ferdinand Enke Verlag.

Coates, T.J., Morin, S.F., & McKusick, L. (1987). Behavioral consequences of AIDS antibody testing among gay men. Journal of the American Medical Association, 258:1889.

Connell, R.W., Crawford, J., Kippax, S., Dowsett, G.W., Baxter, D., & Watson, L. (1989). Facing the epidemic: Changes in the sexual lives of gay and bisexual men in Australia and their implications for AIDS prevention strategies. Social Problems, 36:384-402.

Dannecker, M. (1990). Homosexuelle Männer und AIDS–Eine Sexualwissenschaftliche Studie zu Sexualverhalten und Lebensstil. Schriftenreihe des Bundesministers für Jugend, Familie, Frauen und Gesundheit, Band 252. Stuttgart: Kohlhammer.

Detels, R., English, P., Visscher, B., Jacobson, L., Kingsley, L., Chmiel, J., Dudley, J., Eldred, L., & Ginzburg K. (1989). Seroconversion, sexual activity, and condom use among 2915 HIV seronegative men followed for up to 2 years. Journal of Acquired Immune Deficiency Syndromes, 2:77-83.

Doll, L.S., O'Malley, P., Pershing, A., Hessol, N., Darrow, W., Lifson, A., & Cannon, L. (1988). High-risk behavior and knowledge of HIV-antibody status in the San Francisco City Clinic Cohort. IV International Conference on AIDS, Stockholm, Sverige.

Fox, R., Odaka, N.J., Brookmeyer, R., & Polk, B.F. (1987). Effect of antibody test disclosure on subsequent sexual activity in homosexual men. AIDS, 1:241-246.

Ginzburg, H., Fleming, P., & Miller, K. (1988). Selected public health observations derived from the Multicenter AIDS Cohort Study. Journal of Acquired Immune Deficiency Syndromes, 1:2-7.

Joseph, J.G., Montgomery, S.B., Kessler, R.C., Ostrow, D.G., Wortman, C.B. (1987). Behavioral risk-reduction in a cohort of homosexual men: Two year follow-up. III International Conference on AIDS, Washington DC, USA.

Martin, J. (1987). The Impact of AIDS on Gay Male Sexual Behavior Patterns in New York City. American Journal of Public Health, 77:578-581.

McCusker, J., Stoddard, A.M., Mayer, K.H., Zapka, J., Morrison, J., & Saltzman, S.P. (1988). Effects of HIV antibody test knowledge on subsequent sexual behaviors in a cohort of homosexually active men. American Journal of Public Health 78:462-467.

Niemeck, U., & Schumann, J. (1986). Psychosoziale Auswirkungen von AIDS am Beispiel homosexueller Männer mit und ohne HIV-Antikörper-positiven Befund. Diplomarbeit (Psychologie) Albert-Ludwigs-Universität Freiburg.

Pollak, M. (1990). Homosexuelle Lebenswelten in Zeichnen von AIDS. Soziologie der Epidemie in Frankreich. Ergebnisse Sozialwissenshaftlicher AIDS-Forschubg 4. Berlin: Edition sigma.

Research and Decision Corporation: A report on designing an effective AIDS prevention campaign strategy for San Francisco (1987). Results from the fourth probability sample of an urban gay male community. San Francisco: The San Francisco AIDS Foundation.

Schechter, M., Craib, K., Willoughby, B., Douglas, B., McLeod, A., Maynard, M., Constance, P., & O'Shaughnessy, M. (1988). Patterns of sexual behavior and condom use in a cohort of homosexual men. American Journal of Public Health, 78:1535-1538.

Tillmann, K., Braun, R., Clement, U. (1990). Veränderungen des sexuellen Verhaltens durch die Angst vor AIDS–eine empirische Untersuchung an hetero und homosexuellen Studenten. Öffentliches Gesundheitswesen, 52:323-329.

Van Griensven, G.J.P., Tielman, R.A.P., Goudsmit, J., van der Noordaa, F., de Wolf, F., & Coutinho, R.A. (1987). Effect of HIV-Ab serodiagnosis on sexual behavior in homosexual men in The Netherlands. III. International Conference on AIDS, Washington DC.

Zones, J.S., Beeson, D.R., Echenberg, D.F., Frigo, M.A., O'Malley, P.M., & Rutherford, G.W. (1986). Personal and social consequences of AIDS Antibody testing and notification in a cohort of gay and bisexual man. II. International Conference on AIDS, Paris, Frankrike.

Sexual Aspects of Adaptation
to HIV/AIDS

Susan Schaefer, PhD
Eli Coleman, PhD
Anne-Marie Moore, MC

SUMMARY. Following a pilot study to refine qualitative methods, a phenomenological study consisting of semi-structured interviews with 20 gay men was conducted. The purpose of these interviews was to examine sexuality issues affecting HIV status, both pre- and post-diagnosis. The role of chemical abuse pre-diagnosis emerged as one of the most important factors influencing sexual activity. Following a seropositive HIV diagnosis, significant changes occurred in the sexual behavior of the participants. These changes are outlined in this study along with suggestions made by the participants to resolve potential barriers to healthy sexual functioning. *[Single or multiple copies of this article are available from The Haworth Document Delivery Service: 1-800-342-9678, 9:00 a.m. - 5:00 p.m. (EST).]*

INTRODUCTION

The psychological ramifications of HIV/AIDS present a very complicated clinical picture. Within a relatively short period of time, significant

Susan Schaefer is in private practice in Minneapolis, MN. Eli Coleman is Director and Associate Professor, Program in Human Sexuality, Department of Family Practice and Community Health, University of Minnesota Medical School. Anne-Marie Moore assisted on this project while she was Research Coordinator at the Program in Human Sexuality.

Address correspondence to Eli Coleman, Program in Human Sexuality, University of Minnesota, 1300 South 2nd Street, Suite 180, Minneapolis, MN 55454.

[Haworth co-indexing entry note]: "Sexual Aspects of Adaptation to HIV/AIDS." Schaefer, Susan, Eli Coleman, and Anne-Marie Moore. Co-published simultaneously in *Journal of Psychology & Human Sexuality* (The Haworth Press, Inc.) Vol. 7, No. 1/2, 1995, pp. 59-71; and: *HIV/AIDS and Sexuality* (ed: Michael W. Ross) The Haworth Press, Inc., 1995, pp. 59-71; and: *HIV/AIDS and Sexuality* (ed: Michael W. Ross) Harrington Park Press, an imprint of The Haworth Press, Inc., 1995, pp. 59-71. *[Single or multiple copies of this article are available from The Haworth Document Delivery Service: 1-800-342-9678, 9:00 a.m. - 5:00 p.m. (EST).]*

adjustments are required upon learning of a seropositive diagnosis (Ross, Tebble & Viliunas, 1989). Changes in virtually all major areas of lifestyle are required as the disease progresses. As part of a larger study examining psychological adaptation to HIV/AIDS, this study was designed to identify sexual aspects of adaptation to HIV/AIDS.

With much of the early HIV/AIDS psychological adjustment literature based on anecdotal and clinical reports, the need for systematic studies designed to assess psychological aspects of adaptation to HIV/AIDS was apparent. By studying psychological aspects of adaptation to HIV/AIDS systematically, an attempt was made to circumvent one of the primary criticisms of earlier reports: namely, that findings were based on anecdotal reports alone. As part of a larger study encompassing various adaptations to HIV/AIDS, this study examines the sexual adaptation of gay men after receiving a seropositive diagnosis.

METHODS

Subjects

The charts of 150 patients referred to the HIV Clinic at the University of Minnesota Hospital and Clinics were examined in search of a sample of 20 individuals who fit the criteria guidelines. In order to increase homogeneity of the sample, six selection criteria were applied: (1) self-identified gay males; (2) Caucasian; (3) between the ages of 20-55; (4) diagnosed HIV seropositive; (5) U.S. citizen; (6) high school education or beyond.

Beginning March 1, 1990, the medical charts of all patients who attended the clinic on a regular basis or who presented to the clinic for the first time were reviewed. Once potential subjects who met the aforementioned criteria were identified, they were given a letter of introduction, a brief oral description of the study, and invited to participate. Persons who agreed to take part in the study reviewed and signed an informed consent form. Separate consent forms were used for subjects' degree of participation: personal interview, audiotape, and videotape.

Interview Process

This study was part of a larger study which assessed stressful life events associated with the diagnosis and progression of HIV/AIDS, while also evaluating which types of support were (or would have been) most helpful in managing those stressors. A semi-structured interview, ranging from 1 to 3-1/4 hours in length, was used to gather data. An interview format was chosen over a questionnaire because personal conversations tend to foster rapport building, which in turn increases the likelihood of subjects sharing more deeply, especially in sensitive areas (Jackson and Rothney, 1961; Legacy and Bennett, 1979). The interview was divided into three major portions. Two of the sections tapped information pertaining to demographic/personal background information and recent life changes. Information related to sexual adaptation was included in this part of the interview process.

A pilot study of the initial instrument was conducted with five participants. With the results of this trial procedure, adjustments were made to make the interview as concise, valid, and reliable as possible.

Data Analysis

Qualitative data obtained from the interviews were assessed through thematic content analyses. This reflective abstractive approach (Inhelder and Piaget, 1958) was used to analyze the shared meanings contained in the interviews. This was accomplished through grouping similar statements into content groups and abstracting the information until primary categories were defined and essential meanings (or *meaning units* as they are referred to in phenomenological literature) emerged through the interviewing process. In keeping with Lofland and Lofland's (1984) directive that meanings are best "seen" and analyzed when one assumes a "reality constructionist" stance, this theoretical framework was assumed throughout the research. The reality constructionist stance holds that meanings are not inherent in reality but are imputed by humans.

Giorgi (1989) summarized the essential methodological steps required for qualitative data analysis in this way: (1) reading the material; (2) breaking the material into parts; (3) making sense of the parts through a disciplined or professional way; and (4) reintegration of the parts.

The computer software program *Hyperqual* (Padilla, 1989) was used to systematize this process of qualitative data analysis. This program consists of four stacks which store and organize data derived from interview content. These stacks hold formatted cards which are reproduced as needed to store as much data as a particular interview or collection of interviews generates. Data entered onto these cards, which are identified as meaningful data *chunks,* are highlighted and sent through identifier *buttons* to specific output files. These files become part of an emerging account, constructed by the analyst interacting with the phenomenon under study.

During the preliminary analysis, it is necessary to categorize or codify data. Thematically related text segments can be collated or *chunked* in an output file. Once the analyst is ready to group data chunks together, individual codes called *tags* are attached to the text segments comprising these meaningful data chunks. The data chunks are then sent to new stacks where further refinement of the chunking and coding process takes place. The sorted stacks of text can easily be scanned, called up, and printed out, allowing the analyst to add, change, or delete codes as data chunks are further grouped according to an emerging pattern or account. This software program does not predetermine the process by which data is ultimately analyzed, nor does it require the data to be pre-structured, allowing for maximal flexibility in the data analysis.

RESULTS

Demographics

Participants for this study spanned three decades, ranging in age from 23-53, with 36 being the median age (Table 1). From the sample of 20 men, eight met the criteria for an AIDS diagnosis. Four men were unaware whether or not they met the technical definition guidelines for AIDS. The remaining eight individuals were HIV positive.

Most of the study participants had some technical training or partial college education after completing high school (80%). Occupations were scattered evenly among five categories: service, technical, management, small business owner/operator, and professional. Despite their training, six (30%) participants were supporting themselves through social security

TABLE 1. Participants' Ages

Age Category	Number	Percent
21-25	1	5
26-30	3	15
31-35	4	20
36-40	9	45
41-45	1	5
46-50	0	0
51-55	2	10
Range: 23-53		Median: 36

disability income or other government funding provided for persons with catastrophic illness. Annual income ranged from $4,872 to $50,000, with subsidies for housing, food allowances, and medical care.

The sample was almost equally divided in terms of whether they reported being in a primary relationship (55%) or not (45%). Among the men who were partnered, the average duration of their relationships was six years. Nine (82%) of the eleven partnered men shared a home with their partner. Of the eleven partnered men, nine (82%) reported that they met their partner before they were diagnosed seropositive. Among the partnered subjects, virtually half (55%) of their significant others were also HIV antibody positive. None of the subjects were in relationships with each other.

Substance Use and Abuse

Three quarters (75%) of the men surveyed self-reported periods of substance abuse in their lives, with nine (45%) from the overall sample having received formal treatment for problems arising from their chemical use. It should be noted that this frequency is significantly higher than that routinely reported for gay men in general. Rates of chemical abuse/dependency among gay men typically hover around 33% (Fifield, 1974; Ziebold, 1977), which is dramatically higher than U.S. norms for the general population which are typically reported by the National Institute of Alcohol Abuse and Alcoholism to be 10%.

Chemical abuse and dependency were linked to three particular time periods: college, the coming-out process, and being diagnosed seropositive. The first two periods of drinking and drug use usually occurred within a social context as part of recreational, communal activities. Some of this drug use was normal, while other chemical use which followed the news of testing HIV positive was more abusive in nature, driven by feelings of desperation and appeared to be more of a private, painful activity.

Six (30%) of the men surveyed admitted that their chemical use affected whether or not they practiced safer sex in the past, and a number of others indicated that, although they did not feel it affected their own safe sex practices, they saw it affecting others in the gay community. Some men admitted that when using mood altering chemicals, they often engaged in "compulsive" and/or "reckless" unsafe sex.

Coming-Out Process

Beyond the general demographic data, other important information emerged. Half the men in the sample described their sexual histories as including a rather typical pattern of coming-out as described by Coleman (1981/82). A period of sexual exploration was often followed by serial primary relationships. These men reported a coming-out and exploration period during which time they had frequent sexual contact with numerous persons whom they knew minimally (casual sex) or with whom they were strangers (anonymous sex). Sexual contact with strangers typically occurred at bath houses, bookstores, and parks. This period lasted from months to years and included numerous sexual encounters.

Following this stage, subjects reported they typically became involved in serial partnering which were or were not monogamous, depending on their wishes as well as their partners who often were insistent on maintaining outside liaisons or encouraged the participation in ménage-à-trois or other combinations of multiple sexual partners. Table 2 summarizes the number of sexual partners reported by the sample of gay men. Two thirds of the men (65%) described periods of "compulsive" or "addictive" sex. We did not distinguish how much of this "compulsive" or "addictive" sex was part of a normal developmental process, was "problematic," or symptomatic of a compulsive sexual disorder (see Coleman, 1992 for distinguishing characteristics of compulsive sexual behavior). Three pri-

TABLE 2. Number of Lifetime Sexual Partners

Classification # of Partners	Number (N)	Percent
10-50	5	25
51-100	4	20
101-200	1	5
201-400	1	5
401-800	2	10
801-1,000	1	5
1,001-2,250	1	5
2,251-3,750	2	10
3,751-5,000	1	5
Unable to approximate	2	10
Range: 10-5,000	Median:	288
	Mean:	939
	Projected Mean:	1,021

mary factors were correlated with these periods of compulsive sexual behavior: chemical abuse, acting out linked to anger and/or depression, and sexual activity during the exploration stage of the coming-out process. Approximately 20% of the men had some history of prostitution, ranging from customers to proprietors of gay prostitution businesses.

Safer and Unsafe Sexual Behavior

Prior to their knowledge of being seropositive, a third (35%) of the men shared that they engaged in unsafe sex periodically when they felt down, discouraged, or depressed. When asked, most admitted clearly that these occurrences were conscious, self-destructive acts. A couple of participants were able to identify these experiences as passive suicide attempts.

In comparison to their earlier (pre-seropositive) sexual behavior, seventeen (85%) of the participants reported that their sexual practices took a dramatic shift after being diagnosed seropositive. Four men dealt with their change in HIV status by terminating all sexual activity except self-masturbation. Thirteen (65%) identified their diagnosis as the cutoff point for major shifts in their sexual practices which resulted in more discriminating choices (no further anonymous sex or one night stands), slower, more cautious development towards a sexual relationship, and fewer partners overall.

Since learning of their seropositive status, two-thirds (65%) of the participants stated that they have been completely safe in their sexual practices; a quarter of this group doing so primarily through abstinence. Three men (15%) acknowledged a more gradual development in their safer sex practices, stating it took up to two years to reach a point where safer sex was the norm for them. Another three men (15%) continued to engage in sexual practices which posed some risk, such as eliminating anal sex but continuing oral sex without a condom. The decision to continue sexual practices which posed some risk was based on the consent of their partner and the statistical likelihood of their behavior putting them at risk.

Dimunition of Sexual Interest

Not only did the sexual practices for most of these men markedly change, the importance of sex greatly diminished for the overwhelming majority (70%). Fear of spreading the disease played a role in this diminution, as well as the physical and emotional effects of the disease which left them feeling less sexual. Despite less sexual activity, participants reported gaining a stronger sense of caring, trust, and commitment in their relationships.

The sample was evenly divided as to whether or not they were currently sexually active with a partner. A third of the sample indicated that they were presently sexually active and generally seemed satisfied with their sexual involvement(s). A number of men from this group shared that this came as a surprise to them; at one point in their lives, they couldn't have imagined being content with their present, decreased level of sexual activity. Of those not in a sexual relationship, most did wish to be in a relationship. These men wanted to be sexual but, either due to lack of partner or feeling emotionally shut down, they were not in a sexual relationship.

A number of men commented that their sex drives waned as they became symptomatic. Others were very clear that their own anxieties and fears surrounding potential transmission to a partner (even when practicing safer sex) served to psychologically dampen their sexual desire. As a group, when fears surrounding transmission of the virus interfered with their primary sexual relationships, it was as a result of the fears experienced by the person interviewed as opposed to his partner (45% of whom were not known to be seropositive or who in fact had tested negative).

Two-thirds of the sample (65%) noted decreases in their sexual functioning, as indicated through changes in interest, arousal, and/or ability to perform. These men experienced decreases in the aforementioned areas of sexual functioning. Weighing the many aspects involved, the participants were fairly evenly divided between persons stating they were satisfied with their current sexual activity and those who were not. Those who were sexually satisfied typically (though not always) found themselves prioritizing other aspects of their relationship with a partner, while enjoying less frequent sexual encounters. Among the subgroup who generally were not satisfied with their sexual activity, many were physically or emotionally unable to enjoy sex (either due to fears or physical symptoms).

Barriers Toward Development of a Healthy Sexual Self-Image

As mentioned earlier, a section of the interview tapped the area of sexual relationships, sexual self-image, and sexual difficulties as well as possible obstacles towards the development of a healthy sexual self-image. The prospect of dating after having been diagnosed HIV seropositive carried with it tremendous fears of rejection.

Informing Partners of Their HIV Status. Concerns over how and when to tell a prospective sexual partner about a seropositive diagnosis along with questions of whether it is necessary to say anything at all (especially if one only practices safer sex) were among the most frequent considerations of seropositive persons as they approached dating.

This sample produced quite a range of responses to the question of when (if at all) would they tell a prospective partner of their HIV status. The majority of the group (75%) stressed the importance of telling a partner about their HIV status. They felt it was important to state this early on in the relationship if not immediately.

There was a significant minority (15%) of the participants who felt it was the responsibility of seropositive persons to simply practice safer sex. They maintained that it was not necessary for them to divulge their personal HIV status, viewing this as an invasion of privacy. The remainder of the participants did not have a clear opinion on this matter.

Physical and Psychological Effects of the Disease. Both the physical effects of the disease (e.g., Kaposi's sarcoma lesions) and the psychological ramifications (e.g., fears about transmitting the virus) played significant roles in making the pursuit of a sexual partner more difficult for seropositive persons. Many dealt with their discomfort by abandoning thoughts of actively pursuing a sexual relationship. In an attempt to see what might reverse this tendency, the question was asked "Given your HIV status, what makes pursuing sex with a partner more comfortable for you?" While seventeen (85%) of the subjects were able to pinpoint some specific measures which would definitely contribute to their greater comfort in a dating situation, three individuals were unable to come up with any solutions.

For the former group, the most frequent response centered on knowing that a prospective partner was also HIV positive. Taking time to really get to know a partner before becoming sexually involved was mentioned by a couple participants as important in bringing greater comfort to a dating situation. Additionally, a number of persons felt that interpersonal qualities such as honesty, sincerity, acceptance, and understanding ultimately served to bring the greatest reassurance to a dating experience.

Developing a Healthy Sexual Self-Image

Despite the fact that sexuality was one of the most difficult areas of adjustment for the men studied, when asked what they had learned about engaging in a sexual relationship which may be helpful to others struggling with this issue, a number of important recommendations were made which are summarized with the following statements.

1. "Don't sell short the potential understanding of a prospective sexual partner. Don't automatically assume you cannot or should not be sexual with someone who has tested negative. With informed consent and safe sex practices, this opens up a whole area of relationship possibilities."

2. "Being seropositive certainly does not need to be the end of a sexual relationship. It marks the end of certain aspects of the sexual relationship, but these are things which should also be the case if you are negative. A person who is seropositive can do everything a person who is seronegative can do. You have to adjust it, you don't have to give it up; I never entertain giving up my sexuality."

3. "If you are not having sex after being diagnosed HIV positive, talk about it with others, don't just let it drift away, because it can drift away. One of my best experiences was being in a support group. Someone broke the ice and we all started graphically talking about what we missed. You could feel the healing."

4. "Affirm sex. It is very easy to associate sex with AIDS. Our society is sex negative anyway and more negative towards anything deviating from the norm like homosexuality, making it more difficult to integrate it as something positive. It does seem easy to shift back into sex as bad. Continuing to masturbate, self-pleasuring, this is self-affirmation and a reminder sex can still feel good and be fun. It helps get over fear reactions to orgasm. Being knowledgeable that sex can be safe, not possibly safe but perfectly safe, is important."

5. "It is very important to claim the validity of being a sexual being post HIV. I need to affirm myself that way because at times it feels safer to just not be a sexual being anymore."

6. "Begin the dating process in safe ways. Call an old date (someone safe to start with). Get to know prospective partners as part of larger social group activities first before dating per se."

7. "If you are in a relationship, work it out between the two of you. Don't stop having sex; do whatever you feel comfortable with that is safe."

8. "You have to crash through two closets, that of being gay and that of being seropositive. You have to stay clear of the homophobic messages. You should get involved with support groups, but not just AIDS groups because you can't live it 24 hours. It is important to emphasize living with AIDS rather than dying from AIDS. You need healthy people in your life too, people you can go out and do things with."

9. "Get creative. Write notes to yourself listing what you now can and cannot do. When you come up to a won't, ask yourself why won't you do this; you'll learn something about yourself this way. Tactility is very important, it's a good entree to reclaiming sex, unfreezing what has been shut down. Videos and massage can also help with the unfreezing."

These comments highlight the importance of sexual relationships following a seropositive diagnosis. As mentioned earlier, information about the sexual adaptation of gay men diagnosed with HIV/AIDS was also gathered from a second major section of the interview format–recent life changes. One of the primary goals of this portion of the research was to gather information concerning the major stressors associated with adjustment phases for seropositive persons and to determine what supports received were valuable and what types of support, in retrospect, would have been valuable had it been available. Five specific areas of adjustment were examined: work, financial, family/social, personal, and health.

The Role of Intimate Relationships

Valuable information about the stressful events surrounding family/social issues emerged. Prominent in this section were themes centering on the agony and ecstasy of relationships with others, broken down in fairly distinctive ways. To a very large extent, the primary relationships in these men's lives were incredibly stable given the tremendous numerous stressors they had sustained as a result of dealing with their (and sometimes their partner's) HIV positive status. The relationship with a committed partner was the single most important anchor point and source of solace, comfort, and stability which was described by these men.

DISCUSSION

Significant information about the sexual adaptation of gay men post-seropositive emerged from this qualitative study. However, due to the sample size of 20, any quantitative results should be viewed as general trends or tendencies rather than interpreted as conclusive findings.

Certain phenomena were discovered as gay men made sexual adaptations following a positive HIV-antibody test. The most important transition related to the degree of sexual safety they adopted, as well as the priority placed on sex. Although intimate, homosexual relationships remained meaningful, sexual practices changed dramatically. It appears that the individuals reassessed the sexual risks they were willing to take, while, on a more global level, evaluating the importance of sexuality in relation to other aspects of their lives, often experiencing a shift in priorities.

The results of this study identified obstacles which emerge as HIV-positive gay men attempt to develop a healthy sense of sexuality once diagnosed. Two main issues were identified as impediments: whether or not to inform sexual partners of their HIV status, and the physical and psychological effects of the disease. Combined, these two factors accounted for much of the men's struggle to continue any sexual activity. Concern over informing prospective partners and dealing with the ramifications of the disease process often caused the men to want to avoid dealing with sexuality issues altogether.

This study identified a number of suggestions for HIV-positive individuals wanting to break through these common barriers and engage in sexual relationships. A frequently repeated comment was that sex can still exist, it simply needs to undergo some change. Participants stressed that sex is still important and needs to remain part of one's lifestyle. Related to this was the suggestion to challenge the fears about being sexual; sex must be reaffirmed and validated in spite of the potential risks. The men also recommended that people get to know their potential sexual partners before becoming involved, thus avoiding anonymous sex. Other advice emphasized involvement in support groups as a forum for discussion of fears, concerns, and desires.

Combined with other findings of the larger study (Schaefer, 1992; Schaefer and Coleman, 1992), this study identified the process of sexual adaptation which gay men experience following a diagnosis of HIV. More importantly, it provides insight into the role caregivers and health professionals may play in assisting with the continual process of adaptation.

AUTHOR NOTE

This paper was part of a larger study which was completed by Susan Schaefer as part of the requirements for a Doctoral dissertation at Saybrook University, San Francisco, CA. This research was conducted at the HIV Clinic at the University of Minnesota Hospitals and Clinics.

The authors would like to thank Dr. Frank Rhame, the director of this clinic, for his assistance in helping us identify subjects for this research as well as his helpful suggestions and comments. This research was funded through the HIV Counseling Center which has received funds from the Thorpe Foundation and Mercy Foundation. The authors are most grateful to the participants who volunteered their time, energy, and insight into the psychological processes of their illness.

REFERENCES

Coleman, E. (1981/82). The developmental stages of the coming out process. *Journal of Homosexuality, 7*(2/3), 31-43.
Coleman, E. (1992). Is your patient suffering from compulsive sexual behavior? *Psychiatric Annals, 22*(6), 320-325.

Fifield, L. (1975). *On my way to nowhere: Alienated, isolated, drunk.* Los Angeles Gay Community Services Center Research Project.

Giorgi, A. (1989). Some theoretical and practical issues regarding the psychological phenomenological method. *Saybrook Review, 7*(2), 71-85.

Inhelder, B. and Piaget, J. (1958). *The growth of logical thinking from childhood to adolescence.* New York: Basic Books.

Jackson, R.M. and Rothney, J.W.M. (1961). A comparative study of the mailed questionnaire and the interview in follow-up studies. *Personnel and Guidance Journal, 39,* 569-571.

Legacy, J. and Bennett, F. (1979). A comparison of the mailed questionnaire and personal interview methods of data collection for curriculum development in vocational education. *Journal of Vocational Education Research, 4,* No. 3, 27-39.

Lofland, J. and Lofland, L. (1984). *Analyzing social settings: A guide to qualitative observation and analysis.* Belmont, CA: Wadsworth Publishing Co.

Padilla, Raymond V. (1989). *Hyperqual Software and Users Guide Version 2.0,* Chandler, AZ: Published by the author.

Schaefer, S. (1992). Psychological aspects of adaptation to HIV/AIDS Dissertation Abstracts.

Schaefer, S. and Coleman, E. (1992). Shifts in meaning, purpose, and values following a Diagnosis of Human Immunodeficiency Virus (HIV) Infection Among Gay Men. *Journal of Psychology & Human Sexuality, 5*(1/2), 13-29.

Ross, M.W., Tebble, W.E.M. and Viliunas, D. (1989). Staging of psychological reactions to HIV infection in asymptomatic homosexual men. *Journal of Psychology & Human Sexuality, 2*(1), 93-104.

Ziebold, T. (1977). *Alcoholism and the Gay Community.* Blade Communications, Inc. Washington D.C.

Sexual Dysfunction
in HIV-Seropositive
Women Without AIDS

George R. Brown, MD
Sarah Kendall, PhD
Rebecca Ledsky, MBA

SUMMARY. During a 5.5 year biopsychosocial study, we prospectively assessed the psychiatric status and sexual functioning of women during the natural history of HIV infection (non-AIDS) detected as part of an HIV screening program in the military. Participants were serving on active duty or were spouses of servicemen who have tested HIV-positive since 1986. Patients were psychiatrically evaluated every 6-18 months for three assessments (T1-T3). Initial evaluation (T1) was completed by 54 HIV+ women without AIDS (avg. length of knowledge of seroconversion = 8.9 months). Thirty-eight were reevaluated at T2 (avg. knowledge = 26.5

George R. Brown is Associate Professor of Psychiatry, East Tennessee State University, and Director of Psychiatric Research, Mountain Home VAMC, Johnson City, TN. Sarah Kendall is Research Psychologist, Henry M. Jackson Foundation, San Antonio, TX. Rebecca Ledsky is affiliated with Henry M. Jackson Foundation, Rockville, MD.

Address correspondence to George R. Brown, MD, 175 Bill Jones Road, Jonesborough, TN 37659.

Disclaimer: The views expressed herein are those of the authors and do not necessarily reflect those of the United States Air Force, the Department of Defense, or the Henry M. Jackson Foundation.

[Haworth co-indexing entry note]: "Sexual Dysfunction in HIV-Seropositive Women Without AIDS." Brown, George R., Sarah Kendall, and Rebecca Ledsky. Co-published simultaneously in *Journal of Psychology & Human Sexuality* (The Haworth Press, Inc.) Vol. 7, No. 1/2, 1995, pp. 73-97; and: *HIV/AIDS and Sexuality* (ed: Michael W. Ross) The Haworth Press, Inc., 1995, pp. 73-97; and: *HIV/AIDS and Sexuality* (ed: Michael W. Ross) Harrington Park Press, an imprint of The Haworth Press, Inc., 1995, pp. 73-97. *[Single or multiple copies of this article are available from The Haworth Document Delivery Service: 1-800-342-9678, 9:00 a.m. - 5:00 p.m. (EST).]*

73

months), and 28 at T3 (avg. knowledge = 52.3 months). The most prevalent DSM-III-R psychiatric diagnosis at each evaluation time was Hypoactive Sexual Desire Disorder (HSDD). At T1, 21% met threshold criteria for this diagnosis; an additional 25% had more than a 33% decrease in desire. At T2, 50% had HSDD (new onset in 71% of those women). HSDD was persistently present in 50% at T3 and 50% at T4. A total of 64% (n = 18) were diagnosed with HSDD on at least one visit. Only two women recovered to baseline levels of desire during the time of the study. By the fourth evaluation, 25% of the women seen three times had been pregnant at least once. Twenty-nine percent reported that their male partners actively discouraged their insistence on condom use.

We conclude there is persistent, chronic impairment in sexual functioning in HIV+ women, independent of HIV-related medical symptoms, as reflected in high rates of new onset sexual desire phase disruptions. Potential etiologies are discussed. *[Single or multiple copies of this article are available from The Haworth Document Delivery Service: 1-800-342-9678, 9:00 a.m. - 5:00 p.m. (EST).]*

INTRODUCTION

It is estimated by the World Health Organization that over 2.64 million women are currently infected with the human immunodeficiency virus (HIV) and the rate of new infections in women continues to climb at an alarming rate (CDC, 1993). In the United States alone, over 17,000 women have died of AIDS, accounting for 11% of all deaths in American women 25-44 years old (CDC, 1993). By 1993, heterosexual intercourse was considered the primary mode of transmission for more than 50% of American women with AIDS and up to 80% of those in earlier stages of infection (Brown and Rundell, 1993). Heterosexual transmission has the highest rate of increase of any mode of transmission (CDC, August, 1992). Since the onset of HIV transmission to heterosexual females in the United States (approximately 1979), the percentage of young women 15-19 years of age who report having had sexual intercourse has increased from 42% to 51.5% (including 59% of African-American adolescents; Gayle, 1990). The HIV pandemic is the ever present context within which to consider issues of sexuality and sexual health.

In spite of more than a dozen years of clinical experience with HIV infection in women, few reports on the sexual behavior of infected women are available (Brown and Rundell 1990, 1993; Brown and Pace, 1989; Meyer-Bahlburg et al., 1993) and discussions of sexual health, other than those related to minimizing transmission to uninfected men, are rare. Few researchers have addressed sexual functioning in women living with HIV/ AIDS. Most multicenter cohort studies have not only excluded women but have omitted sexual dysfunctions from diagnostic consideration (Gorman et al., 1991; Ostrow et al., 1989). It has previously been reported that sexual functioning was disrupted in a majority of HIV-seropositive women, with 41% of a group of 29 women evaluated at least twice experiencing hypoactive sexual desire disorder (HSDD) subsequent to learning of seroconversion (Brown and Rundell, 1993). In fact, HSDD was the most common Axis I diagnosis in this group. High proportions (up to 35%) of men and women in our previous cross-sectional study of seropositive persons reported one or more sexual dysfunctions not experienced prior to seroconversion; resolution at one to two years of observation was uncommon (Brown et al., 1992; Brown and Rundell, 1993; Rundell and Brown, 1990).

Expression of sexuality by HIV-infected women is a conundrum. On the one hand, it is the potential "vehicle" of HIV transmission to uninfected partners and infants in utero, while on the other it is the pair-bonding behavior that often plays a crucial role in maintaining intimacy in relationships necessary to the emotional sustenance of both partners. The former has been focused on almost to the complete exclusion of the latter in both the literature and at the International AIDS Conferences. The messages women with HIV often receive from public health authorities, the media, and clinicians is that once infected, sexuality is to be avoided; "sexual health" for HIV-seropositive women is equated with abstinence from interpersonal sexual contact.

Derogatis et al. (1981) previously discussed the psychopathology and symptom profiles of women with and without specific sexual dysfunctions, although Axis I diagnoses were not systematically collected. In this report we present psychiatric diagnostic information in conjunction with sexual behavior data obtained from a group of HIV-seropositive women, none of whom entered the study with AIDS, evaluated longitudinally as part of a 5.5 year prospective study of psychiatric and psychosocial morbidity that began in 1987.

METHODS

The United States Air Force began force-wide, mandatory screenings of all active duty service members for the presence of antibodies to HIV in 1986. Details of the military testing procedure, including safeguards accounting for its exceedingly low rate of false-positive results, are described elsewhere (Burke et al., 1988). All those Air Force personnel confirmed to be seropositive by both ELISA and Western Blot are referred to a single evaluation center (Wilford Hall Medical Center, San Antonio, Texas) for a comprehensive medical, psychiatric, and neuropsychiatric evaluation (Brown et al., 1993). Military medical care beneficiaries (e.g., spouses of airmen) are also eligible for evaluation. Spouses of seropositive active duty personnel are informed, counseled, and offered HIV testing. The psychiatric evaluations for this study were performed by a board certified psychiatrist, senior psychiatric resident, or research psychologist trained in the administration of the Structured Clinical Interview for *DSM-III-R* (SCID; Spitzer et al., 1987). In addition to the structured interview, patients were queried in a semistructured guided interview regarding sexual functioning, sexual behaviors, contraceptive practices, relationship issues, past psychiatric histories, substance use, anxiety and depressive symptoms (SIGH-AD; Williams, 1988) and suicidal ideation (Brown and Rundell, 1990; 1993). Patients returned for reevaluation every 6 to 18 months (dependent upon administrative status, not clinical condition) from their home or base locations throughout the United States, irrespective of whether or not they were retained as active duty members. All interviews were considered epidemiological assessments and were therefore conducted confidentially and not included as part of the military medical record. To further assure confidentiality, research records were identified only by a randomly assigned patient identification number and stored in locked cabinets under the auspices of civilian employees of the Henry M. Jackson Foundation, a nonprofit research organization supporting this work. Both local Institutional Review Board and United States Air Force approval were obtained. Further details of the methodology are provided in an earlier publication (Brown and Rundell, 1993).

The *Diagnostic and Statistical Manual, Third Edition*, Revised (*DSM-III-R*; American Psychiatric Association, 1987) was the source for diagnostic criteria. As objective criteria for diagnosing sexual dysfunctions are lacking in *DSM-III-R* (and, therefore, excluded in the SCID), several of these diagnoses were operationalized for the purposes of this research. These criteria were formulated to emulate the SCID format and were administered at the end of the HIV-version of the SCID interview (Brown et al., 1992; Appendices A and B). For questions regarding relative levels of sexual desire, women served as their own baselines, thereby avoiding the issue of interpreting "desire discrepancies" within couples (Zilbergeld and Ellison, 1980).

Staging of HIV infection was determined by an extensive medical examination previously described (Brown and Rundell, 1993; Brown et al.,

1992) and summarized as a Walter Reed number according to the Walter Reed Classification System (WR) in widespread use throughout the Department of Defense (Redfield et al., 1986). Briefly, stages below WR3 are notable for the presence of greater than 400 T-helper cells/mm3, therefore WR1 and WR2 represent the earliest, usually asymptomatic stages of infection. At the other end of the continuum, WR5 and WR6 are roughly equivalent to CDC-defined Group IV (as applied through 1992; CDC, 1987), consistent with either severe AIDS-related complex (ARC) or AIDS.

Approximately 5% of HIV-seropositive Air Force personnel and dependents evaluated at WHMC since 1987 have been women (women comprise 12.7% of the active duty Air Force). Seventy women were admitted for comprehensive assessment during the course of the study. Sixteen were excluded from analysis on the basis of advanced disease (WR5 or 6) at initial admission (N = 10), nonconsent to participate (N = 1), or admission when the authors were unavailable to enroll them in the study (N = 5). Fifty-four women (89% of those eligible for enrollment) have been evaluated at least once, constituting the T1 evaluation group. Thirty-eight of these patients were evaluated twice (T2), 28 were evaluated three times (T3), 16 were seen four times and 12 were evaluated five times during the 66 month study period. No retrospectively obtained or chart review data were used in this investigation.

A total of 87.1 woman-years of knowledge of HIV-seropositivity were available through the third evaluation time; 138.2 woman-years of knowledge of seroconversion had been logged at the 5.5 year mark, constituting the available experience of living with HIV disease.

Paired statistical comparisons were made between the prevalences of psychiatric diagnoses at T1 and T2, and at T2 and T3 for those women who were evaluated at each of the three time points (fourth and fifth evaluations were excluded from quantitative analysis due to limited sample size). The McNemar test was used in comparisons of these categorical variables (diagnoses) that cannot be assumed to be independent at two points in time (Harris, 1985). The following equation was used in the application of McNemar's test:

$$\text{Chi-square} = \frac{(b-c)^2}{(b + c)}$$

The Wilcoxon rank sum test was used to analyze Hamilton anxiety and depression scale scores. Acceptable type I error was set at $p < .05$.

RESULTS

In general, these women welcomed the opportunity to share information with the examiners and did not express distrust of the confidentiality
safeguards described earlier. The demographic composition of the group at
study entry is described in Table 1. Twenty-six percent (N = 14) of seropositive women reported they were in committed relationships (marriage or
long-term cohabitation) with seropositive male partners at T1. However,
all male partners had not submitted to testing.

Seventy percent of the women evaluated at T1 were seen at T2, with a
minimum of 6 months elapsing between interviews. The average time
between assessments was about 9 months. The racial, marital status, military status, and age composition of the follow-up groups were similar.

Modes of transmission (as assessed by in-depth interview) are listed in
Table 1. As noted, the majority (71%) were likely to have acquired HIV
via unprotected vaginal and/or anal intercourse. Anal intercourse on at
least one occasion any time in the past was reported by six of the T1 group
(two of whom were in the group of 28 seen three times). This sexual
behavior often had to be described by the interviewer as a potential sexual
behavior that "some women participate in" to incredulous study participants before they could respond in the negative. Of the six patients who
reported participation in anal intercourse, only one had engaged in this
activity more than once, and these exposures occurred prior to 1980.

Mode of transmission was unclear or unknown in 11% (N = 6), but
none of these subjects had reported receiving transfusions or using inject-
able drugs.

Seroconversion was noted after a small number of episodes of unprotected vaginal intercourse in 6 women (11%; "low exposure seroconvert-
ers"). For example, a 54 year old black woman with no known CDC-es-
tablished major risk factors who likely became infected after a single
episode of unprotected vaginal intercourse with a known drug user. This
was her only reported sexual encounter since 1979; her male partner later
died of cirrhosis. A second subject, a 21 year old white woman, reported a
total of 10 episodes of intercourse (none involving anal intercourse) with 3
partners and no other risk factors prior to testing positive. A third patient, a
devoutly religious 23 year old pregnant mother of 3 with no known risk
factors and a seronegative husband, reported seroconversion on routine
screening several years after a rape involving a single vaginal exposure.

Our previous work has determined that the length of knowledge of
seroconversion is an important factor in assessing psychiatric morbidity in
HIV-infected populations (Pace et al., 1990; Brown and Rundell, 1993).
At T1, average length of knowledge of seropositivity was 8.9 months

TABLE 1. Characteristics of Patients at Study Entry (N = 54)

Item	N	%
Age		
Youngest	17	
Oldest	59	
Average	28	
Race/Ethnicity		
Caucasian	27	50
African-American	21	39
Hispanic	3	6
Asian	3	6
Marital Status		
Married	35	65
Single/Never Married	15	28
Divorced	4	7
Military Status		
Active Duty	26	48
Dependent	22	40
Retired Military	6	11
Mode of Transmission		
Heterosexual, no known risk group partner(s)	25	46
Heterosexual, high risk or seropositive partner(s)	13	25
Blood Transfusion (pre-1986)	10	19
Intravenous Drug Use	0	0
Indeterminant	6	11
Walter Reed Stage		
1	28	52
2	12	22
3	7	13
4	4	7
5	3	6
CD4 + T Lymphocyte Count		
0-200	4	7
201-500	18	33
>500	32	59

(range 10 days to 43 months; 11.5 months average for the 28 women evaluated three times). Few women were assessed during the turbulent days immediately following notification, and for the purposes of assessing sexual functioning, all such patients were ineligible for a diagnosis of new onset of any sexual dysfunction (see Appendix A). At T2, all women knew of their status for a minimum of one year an average length of knowledge of 26.5 months (range 12.5 to 45 months). Fifty-four percent (N = 20) of women knew of their status for 2 years or more at T2. Average length of knowledge of seroconversion was 52.3 months at T3; 61% (N = 17) had known for at least three years. At T4, 50% (N = 8) had knowingly lived with HIV for at least 4 years.

Selected psychiatric diagnoses relevant to sexual dysfunctions at the first three assessments are listed in Table 2. The first column includes the entire group seen for an initial assessment. The remaining columns are limited to the same group of women evaluated three times to enable direct longitudinal comparisons. Seven women (25%) received a diagnosis of major depressive disorder or dysthymic disorder at one or more visits, although no more than 18% (n = 5) were diagnosed at any one evaluation. A concurrent diagnosis of HSDD was made in three of these subjects during the assessment interval, whereas 15 of 18 women (83%) who were diagnosed with HSDD at one or more visits never met criteria for a mood disorder.

No patients met criteria for inhibited female orgasm or sexual aversion disorder prior to seroconversion by patient report; 4% (N = 2) reported symptoms consistent with lifelong, global HSDD; an additional patient in the T1 group (not reevaluated at T2) noted the insidious onset of this disorder about one year prior to testing positive, but likely to have been after infection occurred. At T1, 48 patients out of the 54 were eligible for the diagnosis of new onset of HSDD since knowledge of seroconversion, since 6 were initially assessed within one month of learning of seroconversion. All patients at T2 and beyond could be assessed for new onset HSDD, as all knew of their serostatus for at least a year. Excluding the two women with lifelong HSDD, a significant increase in those newly diagnosed with HSDD was observed from T1 to T2 (p = .011, McNemar test chi-square = 6.4, df = 1). No additional change from T2 to T3 was observed (p = 1.00, McNemar test). As sexual desire disruptions were by far the most prevalent sexual problems reported, Table 3 lists the changes in desire reported by the participants, using the same definitions for the columns as described above for Table 1. In the first three assessments, no women were diagnosed with sexual aversion disorder (using criteria in Appendix B), hyperactive sexual desire, sexual arousal problems distinct from desire phase disruptions, new onset of inhibited female orgasm, or

TABLE 2. Psychiatric Diagnoses for HIV-Seropositive Women

DIAGNOSIS	T1 (N = 54)	T1 (N = 28)	T2 (N = 28)	T3 (N = 28)
HYPOACTIVE SEXUAL DESIRE DISORDER [a]	13 (24%)	6 (21%)	14 (50%) [b]	14 (50%)
SEXUAL AVERSION DISORDER	0	0	0	0
MAJOR DEPRESSIVE DISORDER	2 (4%)	1 (4%)	2 (7%)	2 (7%)
DYSTHYMIC DISORDER	3 (6%)	1 (4%)	3 (11%)	2 (7%)
GENERALIZED ANXIETY DISORDER	0	0	0	0
ADJUSTMENT DISORDERS	7 (13%)	3 (11%)	1 (4%)	1 (4%)
ALCOHOL DEPENDENCE OR ABUSE	1 (2%)	0	2 (7%)	0
MARITAL PROBLEM	5 (14%)	2 (11%) [c]	6 (30%) [d]	5 (26%) [e]
ANY AXIS II DISORDER	14 (26%)	3 (11%)	5 (18%)	3 (11%)

[a] Lifetime and new onset HSDD since notification of seroconversion
[b] $p = .011$; Chi-square = 6.4, df = 1
[c] N = 19 married
[d] N = 20 married
[e] N = 19 married

81

new abnormalities in the resolution phase of the sexual response cycle. In general, women with low desire who occasionally had intercourse reported normal sexual response phases during sexual activity.

In addition to those who met threshold criteria for HSDD, a significant number of participants reported disruptions in sexual desire and markedly decreased frequencies of sexual activity globally (Table 3).

As a qualitative extension to the data in Table 3, 16 women were reevaluated at T4 (average length of knowledge of seroconversion = 44 months) for sexual dysfunctions. Again, 50% of them (N = 8) had HSDD (including the same 2 patients with lifelong HSDD), and one additional patient developed sexual aversion disorder in the T3-T4 year long interval. This resulted in a 56% prevalence of desire phase disorders at T4. One of the eight patients with HSDD developed this disorder in the T3-T4 interval (length of knowledge >4 years when diagnosed) while two patients with HSDD at T3 no longer met criteria at T4. These two women did not completely resolve their desire disorder, however.

Nine of the 28 women presented with marital problems at one or more evaluations. Six of these (67%) were concurrently diagnosed with HSDD. One third (n = 2) resolved their marital problems in the context of ongoing HSDD, while the remainder did not. Marital problems were noted to increase over time (Table 2). This increase (from 11% of those who were married at T1 to 30% of married couples at T2) followed the same pattern observed for HSDD. Cell sizes were insufficient for meaningful analysis using the McNemar test.

As psychiatric diagnoses are insensitive threshold indicators for some symptoms, Hamilton anxiety (HAM-A) and depression (HAM-D) scale scores were obtained at each visit using the interviewer-administered SIGH-AD (Williams, 1988). Average HAM-A scores were in the subclinical range at each visit (T1: 4.3; T2: 3.6; T3: 4.9). Likewise, average HAM-D scores were low (T1: 4.7; T2: 2.9; T3: 6.1). No women had HAM-A or HAM-D scores in the clinical range (>15) at T1 or T2; 2 subjects scored above 15 on each scale at T3.

To further investigate the relationship between anxiety and depressive symptoms and HSDD, average scores for women with and without HSDD were compared at each visit. Of the six analyses, (T1 to T3 X HAM-A and HAM-D), only HAM-A scores at T1 were significantly higher in those with HSDD compared to those without (8.2 vs. 3.3; p = .039). This relationship was not apparent at subsequent visits, indicating that the symptomatology was largely associated with acute adjustment disorders and/or relatively recent notification of seroconversion.

TABLE 3. Changes in Sexual Desire Reported by HIV-Seropositive Women

PARAMETER	T1 (N = 54)	T1 (N = 28)	T2 (N = 28)	T3 (N = 28)
LIFELONG HSDD	2 (4%)	2 (7%)	2 (7%)	2 (7%)
TOTAL HSDD	13 (27%)[a]	6 (21%)	14 (50%)	14 (50%)
NEW DIAGNOSIS OF HSDD[b]	N/A	4 (14%)	10 (36%)	3 (11%)
HSDD RESOLVED	N/A	N/A	1	3
≥33% DECLINE IN DESIRE (SUBTHRESHOLD FOR HSDD)	10 (19%)	7 (25%)	7 (25%)	2 (7%)
≥33% INCREASE IN DESIRE	0	0	0	0
NO SEXUAL DESIRE[c]	17 (31%)	8 (29%)	5 (18%)	5 (18%)

[a] new onset since previous evaluation
[b] includes all causes, including HSDD
[c] denominator = 48 subjects with ≥ 1 month's knowledge of seropositivity

83

A representative clinical illustration of the new onset of a desire disorder follows.

CASE EXAMPLE, HYPOACTIVE SEXUAL DESIRE DISORDER

A. B., a 27 year old white married woman reported no changes in her sexual desire or functioning within one month after being notified of her HIV seroconversion. Although A. B. was initially quite upset about her seroconversion, it did not surprise her. She was fully evaluated medically and psychiatrically about 6 weeks after her notification. She was completely asymptomatic, had T-cells >500, and no major Axis I disorders. No marital discord was reported. Her husband, also HIV-positive but still asymptomatic and serving on active duty, cared about her a great deal and wanted to continue their previous mutually enjoyable sexual relationship. After about 3-4 weeks, they began to have intercourse again without reported difficulties. At initial assessment, she exhibited no signs or symptoms of HSDD or any other disruption in her sexual functioning (excluding the initial 3-4 week acute adjustment phase when desire was greatly diminished). When reevaluated over a year later, A. B. reported that her sexual drive had gradually, but noticeably, diminished over the past several months to the point where she had "only 10-15% of my normal drive." Her husband was upset by this, and they had begun fighting about "lots of little things." Intimacy in the marriage was significantly impaired, and she wondered if he might have an extramarital affair because of her lack of desire for any type of sex. She did not masturbate, and was not attracted to other men. She scored less than 5 on both Hamilton scales, and no other evidence for a depressive disorder was detected in the course of a two hour interview with the first author. She remained asymptomatic, with T-cells >500, and summarized her own case as: "I'm perfectly fine, I don't have any of those other (physical or psychiatric) symptoms, I love my husband, and I just don't understand why I have lost my desire for sex. This is really upsetting to me." She met our operational criteria for Hypoactive Sexual Desire Disorder, new onset, global, unknown etiology. In addition, a secondary diagnosis of Marital Problem was warranted.

To summarize, A. B.'s case illustrates a number of key features that seemed to present in the majority of the women in this group diagnosed with HSDD:

1. Initial, short term disruption in sexuality after notification of seroconversion (generally one month or less).
2. Insidious onset of decreased sexual desire after resuming sexual activity, including intercourse, with a previous partner (usually her

husband). Decreased drive occurs over months, and is generally upsetting to the woman and/or her partner.

3. Diminished desire usually occurs in the absence of reported physical symptoms or known psychiatric disorders that could readily account for this change.

4. Diminished or absent desire often occurs in the presence of a caring male partner, whether seropositive or seronegative, who wants very much to continue a sexual relationship with her.

5. The woman often cannot explain, or offer any hypotheses for, the genesis of her symptoms.

6. Once established, the severe impairment in sexual desire generally remains chronic and usually does not resolve in those evaluated up to 6 times over a 4-5 year follow up period.

DISCUSSION

Sexual desire involves a complex interplay among intrapsychic, interpersonal, situational, and biological factors. Levine (1988) has dissected the components of desire into sexual drive (spontaneous endogenous arousal, largely based in neuroendocrine mechanisms), wish/aspiration (reflecting self-governance and a sense of appropriateness regarding sexual expression), and motive (consent, or willingness, to behave sexually). He emphasizes that these are reasonably separate entities whose interaction accounts for the end product we understand as "sexual desire." Levine's model implies that disruptions in one or more of these components of desire could result in overall sexual dysfunction. The observation of the new onset of HSDD in a sizeable proportion of the women in this study could therefore be attributable to one or more of the following hypothesized etiologies, each of which will be discussed in turn:

1. Observed prevalences of HSDD are not different from base rates of this disorder in this population.

2. Part of a primary psychiatric or medical condition.

3. Expected concomitant of diagnosis with any life-threatening, probably lethal, condition.

4. Associated with overall stress of adverse life events (HIV-related and otherwise).

5. Direct or indirect influence of HIV on central, hypothalamic and/or neuroendocrine bases of sexual desire.

6. Reflection of negative self-image (including body image).

7. Defense against fear of HIV transmission to others (partners, unborn children).

8. Post-seroconversion disruptions in desire reflect preseroconversion desire phase problems, or a vulnerability to these problems.
9. Guilt and self reproach over sexuality as cause of infection.
10. Anger toward spouse/lover for transmitting HIV to her, sometimes as a result of presumed infidelity.
11. Compliance with societal and medical establishment expectations that HIV-infected women should be both celibate and barren.
12. Multifactorial etiology, both within subjects and for phenomenon as a whole.

Given that this was an uncontrolled study, it is theoretically possible that the high rates of sexual desire problems are not different from what would be observed in any group of Air Force women with similar demographic characteristics. While this cannot be disproved with the data presented here, clinical experience in the military setting is entirely inconsistent with a base rate in excess of 50 percent for sexual dysfunctions, even as a group, in healthy military women. Prevalence rates in nonmilitary clinical samples presenting to sexual dysfunction clinics have been generally similar to that described for this group, e.g., 32% of couples seen by LoPiccolo and Friedman (1988) and 31.7% of married couples reported by Renshaw (1988). Base rates of HSDD in the general population have not been established in a systematic fashion. It is unlikely that the observed, progressive declines in sexual desire in HIV-infected military women reflect a similar phenomenon in the military population at large.

Sexual desire and general physical and psychological well-being are clearly related constructs (Dennerstein et al., 1980). It is well known that anxiety and depression are the most common concomitants of life-threatening disease, e.g., cancer (Andersen, 1985), and disruptions in sexual desire would be expected in this setting. However, the majority of the women in this study were physically asymptomatic, still working or going to school full time, and devoid of significant levels of anxiety or depression with few exceptions. As can be seen in Table 2, diagnoses of mood and anxiety disorders were not common in this group, in contrast to the male sample similarly evaluated at our institution (Brown et al., 1992). Likewise, women with physical symptoms or laboratory evidence associated with advanced HIV disease were initially excluded from participation in this study to further limit the possibility of confounding the results. Further, those who did have clinically relevant anxiety or depressive symptoms received a diagnosis of HSDD on only 3 occasions, whereas HSDD was usually diagnosed in the absence of mood or anxiety disorders (83%). Therefore, the prevalence of HSDD is unlikely to be accounted for by clinically apparent anxiety or depressive disorders in the vast majority of cases.

Women with HIV infection are faced with a number of psychosocial stressors that may contribute to increased levels of stress and, indirectly, to desire phase difficulties. Child-bearing and child-rearing issues ("who will take care of my children after I'm gone?"), loss of jobs, deteriorating quality of life, disclosure of HIV status to friends and family, and obtaining competent health care tailored to their needs are chronic concerns mentioned by women in this study and by others (Kelly et al., 1993; Goldschmidt et al., 1993; Semple et al., 1993). Although the overt effects of these stressors are not always apparent (as evidenced by low rates of depressive and anxiety disorders and generally low Hamilton Anxiety and Depression Scores), such traditional indicators as psychiatric diagnoses and self-report scales may be relatively insensitive measures of the overall levels of stress experienced by these women. Published works examining the stress-moderator model of distress in early HIV infection have focused on numerous potential stress factors and outcomes in men (life events, hardiness, social supports, surrogate markers of disease progression, coping; Goodkin et al., 1992; Blaney et al., 1991; Blomqvist et al., 1991), but sexual functioning outcome parameters in studies of stress in women with HIV disease have not been utilized. Disruptions in sexual desire may be a sentinel marker for the cumulative effects of HIV-related and HIV-independent stressors in otherwise stable, asymptomatic women with early HIV disease.

Women with a known life-threatening diagnosis may exhibit sexual dysfunction in the absence of a primary psychiatric disorder (Schover and Jensen, 1988). A model for comparison may be women with breast or gynecologic malignancies. Women in early stages of breast cancer are generally asymptomatic (except during episodic chemotherapy or radiation treatments), but must live with the notion that they may die prematurely from this disease. The time course for the development of sexual problems in women with breast cancer appears to differ from that observed in women with HIV. For example, longitudinal studies of breast and gynecological cancer patients demonstrate that sexual dysfunctions usually develop early (by 3-4 months) after diagnosis and initial treatment (Andersen, 1987; Vincent, 1975). Up to 50% of these women were diagnosed with one or more sexual dysfunctions in the first 6 months, with a stable or decreasing proportion over the first year (Andersen et al., 1989). By the second year of observation, the number of women developing sexual problems has stabilized, in contrast to that observed in this study, and resolution of sexual dysfunctions over the first year or two was common (Andersen, 1985; Maguire et al., 1978). For women with gynecological malignancies, sexual dysfunction is generally described as more prevalent and severe (Andersen, 1985), with 30% of diagnosed women experiencing one or more dysfunctions at one year follow-up (Andersen et al., 1989). However, if sexual difficulties did arise in women with gynecologic cancers, they generally presented early, as soon as intercourse was attempted, not as a later onset, insidious process after a period of adequate functioning (Andersen et al., 1989).

The sexual "drive" component of sexual desire is largely accounted for by neuroendocrine mechanisms (Levine, 1988). The linkage between female sexual desire and testosterone levels has been explored, with suggestive results from correlational studies (Segraves, 1988). Two studies have shown a positive correlation between circulating free testosterone levels and frequency or enjoyment of sexual interaction with a partner (Persky et al., 1982; Morris et al., 1987). Unfortunately, this neuroendocrine hypothesis was suggested post hoc, and measures of free testosterone were not obtained in their participants. Assessments of reproductive hormones in HIV-infected women have been reported only once to our knowledge (Shah et al., 1993), and testosterone was excluded from consideration. Testosterone levels were available only for two patients with new onset HSDD in this study, with one low result (10 ng/dl) and one in the normal female range (60 ng/dl; reference range 25-95 ng/dl). Decreased limbic sensitivity to testosterone has been hypothesized as an etiology of decreased desire in the elderly. As HIV ultimately causes dementia in a large percentage of AIDS patients, it is possible that HIV accelerates an aging process that results in premature loss of sensitivity to circulating testosterone which is, after all, normally present only in minute quantities in women of any age. This remains highly speculative, as currently available data from HIV-infected patients cannot adequately address the contributions, if any, of neuroendocrine abnormalities in women with disrupted sexual desire.

Some women at one or more evaluation times suffered from negative self-image and, specifically, negative body image. They reported feeling "dirty," "diseased," "untouchable," or "unlovable" because of their infection. Impaired sexuality would be a concomitant for these women, although this dynamic was neither consistently present in individual cases nor apparent in more than several women at any evaluation time.

More common was the concern over transmitting HIV to either an unborn baby or to a seronegative male partner. This was the primary reason given by women when asked to "autognose" their sexual dysfunction. Some expressed fear, rather than concern, over this possibility, especially in light of the fact that 29% of the women reported that their husband or lover had tried to dissuade them from using a condom on one or more occasions (even if her partner was seronegative). Although this concern is well placed, a conscious decision to eliminate transmission risk should not eliminate sexual desire *per se* or the ability to engage in safe alternatives to intercourse or self-stimulation. Women who provided this explanation rarely engaged in these alternatives and had global impairment of desire in all settings. Thus, although this explanation seems plausible on the surface, the link between a conscious desire to protect others and chronic, global, late(r) onset desire phase disorders is unclear.

The observations in this longitudinal study are consistent with the concept of preseroconversion vulnerability to sexual dysfunction in women who ultimately become infected. In our parallel study of men with early HIV infection, comparisons to available community comparison groups indicated that military men who eventually became infected had a higher than expected lifetime (preseroconversion) incidence of depressive disorders as well as a significantly elevated prevalence of mood disorders after notification of seroconversion (Brown et al., 1992). Although hypotheses for this phenomenon in HIV-infected men are commonly generated (e.g., the stress of living a closeted life as a gay or bisexual man in the military may predispose such men to substance use disorders and mood disorders, irrespective of HIV status), the social issues for women in the military setting are markedly different and do not readily account for preseroconversion vulnerability to sexual desire disorders. The fact that only two women in this study reported a history consistent with a preseroconversion sexual dysfunction further calls this proposed etiology into question.

Guilt and self-reproach over sex as the root cause of their infection (in up to 81%) could be responsible for the development of desire disorders in some of the women interviewed. One woman stated that "sex is the farthest thing from my mind now; it's what got me into this mess in the first place." Some women reported that they consciously isolated themselves socially to avoid any potential encounters with men that could lead to a sexual relationship. Two women who felt guilty over their "stupidity" in not protecting themselves during intercourse chose to deal with their self-reproach by becoming public speakers in high schools and elsewhere, relating their personal experiences in hopes of reaching other women who are at risk.

As noted by Levine (1988, p. 31), "the presence of sexual desire implies an acknowledgement that, all things considered, the relationship outside the bedroom is acceptable." Such was clearly not the case in some of the relationships in this sample. Anger toward their male partner, consciously expressed or unconsciously repressed, could result in diminished desire for sexual intimacy in some of the women in this study. This was suggested by two women who reported that their spouses had likely been unfaithful to them and "brought it (HIV) home." Most are aware that transmission from men to women in the U.S. is many times more likely than vice versa (Padian et al., 1991) and assumed they were victims of their partner's infidelity. Decreased desire would therefore be more of an expression of an active, strong desire **not** to have sex with their partner than a passive lack of desire. This explanation should result in early onset of limited, partner-specific HSDD rather than the global form of HSDD observed in the participants, although no women reported limited or partner-specific desire problems.

Increasing marital problems in those who were married appeared to be both a product of and an antecedent to disruptions in sexual desire. Husbands universally wanted to remain sexually active with their wives, irrespective of their own HIV serostatus. This was true even into late stage disease for the men, according to their wives' reports. The lack of desire for sexual contact of any type significantly altered the sexual equilibrium previously established in their relationship, resulting in anger, disappointment, and, at times, threats on the part of the men. A positive feedback loop was established, wherein continuing lack of sexual desire contributed to further deterioration of marital intimacy, and general relationship deterioration contributed to, or more likely maintained, disrupted sexual desire in the HIV-positive women.

Impaired sexual desire in HIV-seropositive women is consistent with the prevailing bias in our society, particularly in the medical community, that HIV-infected women should no longer behave sexually. The experience of some of the women in this study who sought prenatal care or obstetric services (25% of the cohort had been pregnant at least once while HIV-seropositive) was one of disdain and overwhelming negativism toward their consideration of childbearing. Routine gynecological exams for some of those who were not pregnant were described as "gown and glove circuses"; dental care was impossible to obtain by women in some rural communities. The messages they received from health care providers, military commands, and public health sources were unambiguously sex-negative and in the service of abstinence from sexual expression. The "benefit" of decreased or absent sexual desire is that these issues become moot, enabling the women to unconsciously "trade" her sexual life for greater social acceptance and less derision. This potential sociological etiology merits further consideration.

As in many complex psychosexual phenomena, a multiply determined process is the most likely explanation for sexual dysfunction in the majority of the women interviewed. Although several of the proposed hypotheses appear unlikely as individual determinants, a combination of two or more could account for the findings. For example, a decrease in key neuroendocrine levels (but remaining in the acceptable, "normal" range) in combination with psychosocial factors (anger, guilt, low self-esteem) or stressors (caring for HIV-infected family members, loss of job, financial hardship) seems a plausible, albeit unproven multifactorial etiology. What is clear, however, is that the "dynamic nature of sexuality and its complex interplay with biopsychosocial events makes it imperative to study the disease-sexuality interface longitudinally, not cross-sectionally" (Andersen et al., 1989). This approach has, at the very least, enabled us to propose the likely candidates that help us understand the sexual problems experienced by women with HIV disease.

In addition to diminishing quality of life, the development of HSDD has potential implications for HIV disease transmission as well. Marital discord was observed to increase after the first evaluation to 30% of the married couples. Wives with desire phase disorders mentioned the pivotal role of their global lack of interest in sexual contact in the deterioration of their marriages, since their husbands uniformly wanted to continue intercourse irrespective of their own serostatus. Some have voiced concern that their partners may seek or become vulnerable to extramarital affairs as a result of their dysfunction. It is possible that this is more than an idle concern, resulting in higher rates of extramarital sexual activity fueled by increasing marital discord and decreasing intimacy in their relationship with an infected woman with sexual desire problems.

The observations in this study suggest a number of areas for future study. Partners of HIV-infected women could provide important insights into sexual dysfunctions in their relationships beyond what can be gleaned from an assessment of the women alone. No partners were systematically interviewed for this study, largely because the women were usually flown to San Antonio from around the country for their ongoing HIV assessments in the absence of their partner. We are unaware of any studies that have explored the effects of HIV on the sexual relationships of women infected with HIV from the perspective of their male, or female, partners. Also, neuroendocrine studies could be very useful in understanding the etiology of this condition, as noted above, and could lead to potential treatment considerations.

Last, it is not known whether traditional sex therapy techniques would be helpful in this population. Global HSDD in women is traditionally considered one of the most difficult sexual dysfunctions to treat by any known methods, due in part to its multiply determined and poorly understood etiologies (Kaplan, 1977; Vandereycken, 1987). Improving the quality of life for women living with HIV/AIDS through sensitively addressing this problem and systematically studying potential treatments is warranted.

The results of this study need to be considered in the context of its limitations. Although this is the largest study published to date examining sexual functioning in a prospective fashion in women with early stage HIV disease, the sample size is still small. Further, the observations described here may not apply to other populations [e.g., the inner city, injecting drug using sample reported by Meyer-Bahlburg and associates from New York City (Meyer-Bahlburg et al., 1993)], or to women with AIDS. Important demographic differences exist between this sample and the U.S. population of women with AIDS, recently characterized as 74% African-American or Hispanic and comprising at least 50% with significant injecting drug use experience (CDC, August, 1992). Last, the formal diagnosis of HSDD (and most other sexual dysfunctions) traditionally involves clinical judgement applied to the context of an individuals' and couples' lives; standardized and quantifiable criteria are not well established. Therefore, although we attempted to operationalize the *DSM-III-R* criteria for some sexual dysfunctions, it is possible that our listed prevalences do not accurately reflect the true prevalences of these conditions.

CONCLUSION

In conclusion, our observations indicate that disruptions in the desire phase of the sexual response cycle are not only prevalent in women with HIV, but increase over at least the first year or more after notification of seroconversion. This increase is observed both in the formal diagnosis of HSDD and in the proportion of women who report subthreshold levels of disruptions in baseline levels of desire. A plateau in the rate of development of HSDD appears to be reached by the second assessment (after 18-24 months of knowledge of seropositivity) with between 50%-56% of women reaching threshold criteria for a desire phase disorder (64% diagnosed with HSDD at least once). Some women improve when followed for 3-5 years, but complete resolution of the symptoms was rare. Simple associations with physical illness or comorbid psychiatric conditions do not appear to account for these observations. HIV-related changes in neuroendocrine mechanisms that serve as a substrate for the drive component of female sexual desire could be involved. Although etiology in most cases is unknown, it is most likely to be multifactorial. Levine's (1988) model of the tripartite nature of sexual desire (drive, wish, motivation) may be a useful construct in addressing the complexities observed. We agree with Meyer-Bahlburg and colleagues (1993) that routine assessments of the ever-increasing population of HIV-seropositive women should include questions about sexual health and functioning, along with standard evaluations of gynecological, medical, and mental health. Women living with HIV/AIDS need to be viewed as people with very real needs for intimacy that may reasonably include responsible sexual contact with others, not just as 'vectors of transmission' to men and infants. Helping professionals caring for these women can better serve their mental health needs if they are able to deliver the message that sexual health for those living with HIV/AIDS is not simply equated with abstinence.

AUTHOR NOTE

The authors warmly thank Billy Stinnett for extensive assistance with data analysis and table preparation. John Kozjak, and Dorothy Haas provided invaluable assistance in the recruitment, and administration phases of this work. Robert Zachary, PhD, Heino Meyer-Bahlburg, Dr. rer. nat., and Karen Washington, MSM provided helpful comments on the manuscript. The authors especially thank the military women who shared the intimate details of their lives to make this work possible. This work was supported, in part, by a grant administered by the Henry M. Jackson Foundation for the Advancement of Military Medicine.

REFERENCES

American Psychiatric Association (1987). Diagnostic and Statistical Manual of Mental Disorders, Third Edition, Revised. Washington, D.C., American Psychiatric Association Press.

Andersen B (1985). Sexual functioning morbidity among cancer survivors. Cancer 55:1835-1842.

Andersen B (1987). Sexual functioning complications in women with gynecologic cancer. Cancer 60:2123-2128.

Andersen B, Anderson B, deProsse C (1989). Controlled prospective longitudinal study of women with cancer: I. Sexual functioning outcomes. Journal of Consulting and Clinical Psychology 57:683-691.

Blaney N, Goodkin K, Morgan R, Feaster D, Millon C, Szapocznik J, Eisdorfer C (1991). A stress-moderator model of distress in early HIV-1 infection: Concurrent analysis of life events, hardiness, and social support. Journal of Psychosomatic Research 35:297-305.

Blomqvist V, Jonsson L, Töres T (1991). Life events and coping patterns reported in HIV-infected hemophiliacs a year after diagnosis. Scandinavian Journal of Social Medicine 19:94-98.

Brown G, Pace J (1989). Reduced sexual activity in HIV-infected homosexual men. Journal of the American Medical Association 261:2503-2504.

Brown G R, Rundell J R (1990). Prospective study of psychiatric morbidity in HIV-seropositive women without AIDS. General Hospital Psychiatry 12:30-35.

Brown G, Rundell R (1993). Prospective study of psychiatric aspects of early HIV disease in women. General Hospital Psychiatry 15:139-147.

Brown G R, Rundell J, McManis S, Kendall S, Zachary R, Temoshok L (1992). Prevalence of psychiatric disorders in early stages of HIV infection in United States Air Force Personnel. Psychosomatic Medicine 54:588-601.

Brown G R, Rundell J, McManis S, Kendall S, Jenkins R (1993). Neuropsychiatric morbidity in early HIV disease: Implications for military occupational function. Vaccine 11(5):560-569.

Burke D, Brandage J, Redfield R et al. (1988). Measurement of the false positive rate in a screening program for human immunodeficiency virus infections. New England Journal of Medicine 319:961-964.

Centers for Disease Control (1987). Revision of the CDC surveillance case definition for acquired immunodeficiency syndrome. Morbidity and Mortality Weekly Report 36:1-15.

Centers for Disease Control (1990). AIDS in women: United States. Morbidity and Mortality Weekly Report 39:845.

Centers for Disease Control (1992, August). HIV/AIDS prevention: Facts about women and HIV/AIDS. Atlanta.

Centers for Disease Control (1993). Update: Mortality attributable to HIV infection/AIDS among persons aged 25-44 years-U.S., 1990 and 1991. Morbidity and Mortality Weekly Report 42:481-486.

Dennerstein L, Burrows G, Wood C, Hyman G (1980). Hormones and sexuality: Effect of estrogen and progesterone. Obstetrics and Gynecology 18:139-143.

Derogatis L (1980). Breast and gynecologic cancers: Their unique impact on body image and sexual identity in women. In: Vaeth JM, ed. Frontiers of Radiation Therapy and Oncology, Vol. 14. Basel: S Karger AG, Basel, pp. 1-11.

Derogatis L, Meyer J, King K (1981). Psychopathology in individuals with sexual dysfunction. American Journal of Psychiatry 138:757-763.

Gayle J (1990). Surveillance for AIDS and HIV infection among black and hispanic children of childbearing age, 1981-1989. In CDC Surveillance Summaries, July 1990. Morbidity and Mortality Weekly Report 39 (No. 55-3):23-30.

Goldschmidt M, Temoshok L, Brown G R (1993). Women and HIV/AIDS. In *The Health Psychology of Women*, Harwood Academic Publishers, London.

Goodkin K, Fuchs I, Feaster D, Leeka J, Rishel D (1992). Life stressors and coping style are associated with immune measures in HIV-1 infection—A preliminary report. International Journal of Psychiatry in Medicine 22:155-172.

Gorman J, Kertzner R, Todak G et al. (1991). Multidisciplinary baseline assessments of homosexual men with and without human immunodeficiency virus infection. I. Overview of study design. Archives of General Psychiatry 48:120-123.

Harris R (1985). A Primer of Multivariate Statistics. Orlando, FL, Academic Press.

Kaplan H (1977). Hypoactive sexual desire. Journal of Sex and Marital Therapy. 3:3-9.

Kelly P, Holman S, Ehrlich I, Driscoll B, Chirgwin K, DeHovitz J (1993). Quality of life measurement in HIV positive women. Proceedings of the 9th International AIDS Conference, Berlin, Germany, PO-B32-2266.

Levine S (1988). Intrapsychic and individual aspects of sexual desire. In Leiblum S, and Rosen R (Eds.), Sexual Desire Disorders, Guilford, New York, pp. 21-44.

LoPiccolo J, Friedman J (1988). Broad-spectrum treatment of low sexual desire: Integration of cognitive, behavioral, and systematic therapy. In Leiblum S, and Rosen R (Eds.), Sexual Desire Disorders, Guilford, New York, pp. 107-144.

Maguire G, Lee E, Bevington D, Kuchemann C, Crabtree R, Cornell C (1978). Psychiatric problems in the first year after mastectomy. British Medical Journal 1:963-965.

Meyer-Bahlburg H, Nostlinger C, Exner T, Ehrhardt A, Gruen R, Lorenz G, Gorman J, El-Sadr W, Sorrell S (1993). Sexual functioning in HIV+ and HIV − injected drug-using women. Journal of Sex and Marital Therapy 19:56-68.

Morris N, Udry J, Khan-Dawood F, Dawood M (1987). Marital sex frequency and midcycle female testosterone. Archives of Sexual Behavior 16:147-157.

Ostrow D, Monjan A, Joseph J et al. (1989). HIV-related symptoms and psychological functioning in a cohort of homosexual men. American Journal of Psychiatry 146:737-742.

Pace J, Brown G, Rundell J, Paolucci S, Drexler K, McManis S (1990). Prevalence of psychiatric disorders in a mandatory screening program for infection with human immunodeficiency virus: A pilot study. Military Medicine 155:76-80.

Padian N, Shiboski S, Jewell N (1991). Female-to-male transmission of human immunodeficiency virus. Journal of the American Medical Association 266:1664-1667.

Persky H, Dresibach L, Miller W, O'Brien C, Khan M, Lief H, Charnery N, and Strauss D (1982). The relation of plasma androgen levels to sexual behaviour and attitudes of women. Psychosomatic Medicine 44:305-319.

Redfield R, Wright D, Tramont E (1986). The Walter Reed staging classification for HTLV-III/LAV infection. New England Journal of Medicine 314:131-132.

Renshaw D (1988). Profile of 2376 patients treated at Loyola Sex Clinic between 1972 and 1987. Sex and Marital Therapy 3:111-117.

Rundell J, Brown G R (1990). Persistence of psychiatric symptoms in HIV-seropositive persons. American Journal of Psychiatry 147:674-675.

Schover L, Jensen S (1988). Sexuality Problems and Chronic Disease: A Comprehensive Approach, Guilford Press, New York.

Segraves R (1988). Hormones and libido. In: Sexual Desire Disorders, Leiblum S and Rosen R (eds.), Guilford, New York.

Semple S, Patterson T, Temoshok L, McCutchan J, Straits-Tröster K, Chandler J,

Grant I et al. (1993). Identification of psychobiological stressors among HIV-positive women. Women & Health 20(4):15-36.

Shah P, Smith J, Wells C, Iatrakis G, Barton S, Kitchen S (1993). Endocrine function in HIV seropositive women: A case controlled study. Proceedings of the 9th International AIDS Conference, Berlin, Germany, PO-B25-1964.

Spitzer R, Williams J, Gibbon M, First M (1987). Structured Clinical Interview for DSM-III-R (SCID). New York, NY: Biometrics Research Division, New York State Psychiatric Institute.

Vandereycken W (1987). On desire, excitement, and impotence in modern sex therapy. Psychotherapy and Psychosomatics, 47:175-180.

Vincent C, Vincent B, Greiss F, Linton E (1975). Some marital-sexual concomitants of carcinoma of the cervix. Southern Medical Journal 68:552-558.

Williams J (1988). The Structured Interview Guide for the Hamilton Depression and Anxiety Scales. Biometrics Research Department, New York State Psychiatric Institute, New York, NY.

Zilbergeld B, Ellison C (1980). Desire discrepancies and arousal problems in sex therapy. In S. Leiblum & L. Pervin (Eds.), Principles and Practice of Sex Therapy, New York, Guilford Press.

APPENDIX A

OPERATIONAL CRITERIA FOR THE DIAGNOSIS OF HYPOACTIVE SEXUAL DESIRE DISORDER IN HIV-SEROPOSITIVE PERSONS*

A. Persistently or recurrently deficient or absent sexual fantasies and desire for sexual activity of any type.

B. If new onset of diminished desire can be identified, the subjective amount of desire is rated as at least one third less than the individual's baseline level.

C. The disturbance in sexual desire must be present continuously for at least one month.

D. At least one month has passed since the patient was notified of HIV seropositive status.

E. The disturbance causes distress or interpersonal difficulties.

F. Does not occur exclusively in the context of sexual aversion disorder or another major Axis I diagnosis; may be concurrently diagnosed in the presence of relevant V-code diagnoses or other sexual dysfunctions.

G. It cannot be established that an Axis III condition (primary medical disorder) or other organic factor initiated and maintained the disturbance.

SPECIFY ETIOLOGY:	Psychogenic only or Combined Bio-genic and Psychogenic
SPECIFY CHRONOLOGY:	Lifelong deficient or absent desire Acquired deficit since HIV sero-conversion Acquired prior to, or apparently unrelated to seroconversion
SPECIFY CIRCUMSTANCES:	Limited to certain partner(s) or Gen-eralized

*The structured interview format for Hypoactive Sexual Desire Disorder and Sexual Aversion Disorder is available from the author.

APPENDIX B

CRITERIA FOR DIAGNOSIS OF SEXUAL AVERSION DISORDER IN HIV-SEROPOSITIVE PERSONS*

A. Persistent or recurrent aversion to, and avoidance of, all or almost all, genital sexual contact with a sexual partner.
B. The disturbance must be present more often than not for at least a one month duration.
C. Does not occur exclusively in the context of another major Axis I diagnosis; may be concurrently diagnosed in the presence of relevant V-code diagnoses or other sexual dysfunctions with the exception of hypoactive sexual desire disorder.
E. It cannot be established that an Axis III condition or other organic factor initiated and maintained the disturbance.

SPECIFY ETIOLOGY:	Psychogenic only or Combined Bio-genic and Psychogenic
SPECIFY CHRONOLOGY:	Lifelong deficient or absent desire Acquired deficit since HIV sero-conversion Acquired prior to, or apparently unrelated to seroconversion
SPECIFY CIRCUMSTANCES:	Limited to certain partner(s) or Gen-eralized

*The structured interview format using these criteria is available from the authors.

Sexual Risk Behavior Among Women with Injected Drug Use Histories

Anke A. Ehrhardt, PhD
Christiana Nöstlinger, PhD
Heino F. L. Meyer-Bahlburg, Dr. rer. nat.
Theresa M. Exner, PhD
Rhoda S. Gruen, MA
Sandra L. Yingling, MA
Jack M. Gorman, MD
Wafaa El-Sadr, MD
Stephan J. Sorrell, MD

SUMMARY. This study documents the sexual risk behavior for HIV infection and transmission in inner-city women with a history of injected drug use (IDU). The sample consists of N = 38 HIV+ and N = 37 HIV − women who were demographically comparable. A surprisingly high number of women in both groups reported both

Anke A. Ehrhardt, Heino F. L. Meyer-Bahlburg, Theresa M. Exner, Rhoda S. Gruen, Sandra L. Yingling, and Jack M. Gorman are all affiliated with the HIV Center for Clinical and Behavioral Studies at New York State Psychiatric Institute and Columbia University, New York, NY; Christiana Nöstlinger is affiliated with Harlem Hospital Center, New York, NY; and Wafaa El-Sadr and Stephan J. Sorrell are affiliated with St. Luke's/Roosevelt Hospital Center, New York, NY.

Address correspondence to Dr. Ehrhardt at New York State Psychiatric Institute, Unit 10, 722 West 168th Street, New York, NY 10032.

Supported by Grant 5-P50-MH43520 from NIMH/NIDA to the HIV Center for Clinical and Behavioral Studies and Training Grant 5-T32-MH19139 from NIMH.

[Haworth co-indexing entry note]: "Sexual Risk Behavior Among Women with Injected Drug Use Histories." Ehrhardt, Anke A. et al. Co-published simultaneously in *Journal of Psychology & Human Sexuality* (The Haworth Press, Inc.) Vol. 7, No. 1/2, 1995, pp. 99-119; and: *HIV/AIDS and Sexuality* (ed: Michael W. Ross) The Haworth Press, Inc., 1995, pp. 99-119; and: *HIV/AIDS and Sexuality* (ed: Michael W. Ross) Harrington Park Press, an imprint of The Haworth Press, Inc., 1995, pp. 99-119. *[Single or multiple copies of this article are available from The Haworth Document Delivery Service: 1-800-342-9678, 9:00 a.m. - 5:00 p.m. (EST).]*

male and female sex partners during their lifetime, and significantly more HIV+ women currently identified as bisexual and lesbian. Overall, HIV+ women had had more lifetime male and female sex partners, although the two groups did not differ in their current sexual behavior regarding numbers of partners and sex occasions. Both groups of women had little information about risk characteristics of their male sex partners, except for a history of IDU that was common among partners of both HIV+ and HIV − women. Sex for money was practiced by a subgroup of women in both groups and sex in exchange for drugs by very few women. A disturbingly high number of HIV+ and HIV − women reported occasions of unprotected sex during the past six months (86% vs. 97%), a finding that suggests that educational efforts for behavior change in IDU women need to be intensified. *[Single or multiple copies of this article are available from The Haworth Document Delivery Service: 1-800-342-9678, 9:00 a.m. - 5:00 p.m. (EST).]*

INTRODUCTION

Women with a history of injected drug use (IDU) currently compose the largest category of AIDS cases among adult women in the United States (Centers for Disease Control [CDC], 1992). Little is known about the sexual behavior of these IDU women. Unlike IDU men, whose primary sexual relationships tend to be with women who do not themselves inject drugs, IDU women are apt to be partnered with IDU men (Turner, Miller, and Moses, 1989), placing them at double risk related to drug use: their own needle-sharing behavior and sex with a high-risk partner. Although needle sharing is a highly efficient mode of HIV transmission and a likely route of HIV infection for many IDUs, it is unclear for how many it was their sexual behavior with an infected partner that caused infection.

Overall, heterosexual transmission among women is increasing. In the U.S., the percentage of women with AIDS who were infected through heterosexual transmission grew from 13% in 1982 to 34% by March 1992, while the proportion exposed through injected drug use remained relatively stable at 50% (CDC, 1992). In the past, research has focused particularly on the drug use risk behavior of IDUs rather than on their sexual behavior, but there is evidence that needle-sharing behavior among IDUs has declined from approximately 46% in 1984 to 14% in 1988, while sexual risk behavior has remained relatively unchanged (Battjes and Pickens, 1988; Harris, Langrod, and Hebert, 1990).

Thus, the study of sexual risk behavior of HIV-positive (HIV+) women and of comparable groups of HIV-negative (HIV −) women is timely and important for several reasons: (1) detailed assessment of sexual risk behavior is necessary if effective interventions are to be developed; (2) the comparison of the sexual histories of HIV+ and HIV− women may give us insight into the likely risk factors that were responsible for seroconversion; and (3) repeated assessments of sexual risk behavior in HIV+ women may identify factors that contribute to disease progression and that may be indicators for treatment strategies.

The purpose of this paper is to describe the sexual risk behaviors among a New York City cohort of HIV+ and HIV− women with a history of IDU. Their behaviors were assessed at baseline and at six-month intervals as part of a prospective longitudinal study. This paper will focus on the baseline assessment only and will address sexual risk factors such as partner frequency, sexual practices, sex for money and drugs, and partner risk indicators. We will also report on differences and similarities between the HIV+ and HIV− women and will thus explore the role of HIV seropositivity on sexual risk behavior among IDU women.

METHODS

Sample Selection

Seventy-five women with a history of IDU were recruited from two New York City sites. The majority were recruited through advertisements at various institutions in Harlem and through referrals and word-of-mouth within the drug-abusing community; the remainder were from a methadone clinic at Roosevelt Hospital. The inclusion criteria were: for the Harlem sample, injected drug use at least ten times since 1982 and at least once in the preceding 12 months, and for the Roosevelt Hospital sample, attendance at the methadone maintenance program for at least three months and use of injected drugs at least ten times since 1982, but not necessarily in the preceding 12 months. All the women were required to know whether their HIV status was positive or negative prior to entry in the study. Their HIV status was subsequently confirmed by replication of HIV testing. Since the goal was to recruit women at a relatively asymptomatic stage of HIV disease, women who, at baseline, met the CDC criteria for AIDS were excluded. All participating women had to be able to speak and understand English. The resulting cohort comprised 38 HIV+ and 37 HIV− women.

Assessment

Each woman participating in the study received a comprehensive evaluation including medical, neurological, neuropsychological, psychiatric, psychosocial, and psychosexual assessments. Sexual behavior and functioning were evaluated at baseline by the Sexual Risk Behavior Assessment Schedule–Adult, Baseline Interview for Female Drug Users [SERBAS-A-DF-1] (Meyer-Bahlburg, Ehrhardt, Exner, Calderwood, and Gruen, 1988). The SERBAS-A-DF-1 is a semi-structured interview schedule designed to cover sexual risk behavior and dysfunctions during the six months prior to the interview, as well as to elicit information on "lifetime" sexual activity. This interview has been derived in part from the Sexual Behavior Assessment Schedule–Adult [SEBAS-A] (Meyer-Bahlburg and Ehrhardt, 1983). (For further details about the SERBAS-A, see Meyer-Bahlburg, Exner, Lorenz, Gruen, and Gorman, 1991.)

The interview language was modified to be appropriate for the women of the study, and the content was adapted for the purposes of the current project. A retest reliability study (unpublished data) of the SERBAS-A-DF-1 in this population showed good reliability for reports of sexual behavior for the six months prior to interview. The interview took approximately one hour to complete.

Interviewers were masters-level clinicians who were extensively trained with a standard protocol (Gruen and Meyer-Bahlburg, 1992) in the use of the SERBAS-A-DF-1. With the rare exception of an individual refusing audiotaping, all interviews were taped. The interviews were subsequently scanned for internal consistency and completeness, and attempts were made to resolve any inconsistencies with the assistance of tape recordings and interviewer consultations. The training supervisor monitored interviewer performance throughout the study by reviewing at least every seventh interview, and this was followed by individual feedback and weekly group supervision sessions.

The risk-behavior section of this interview uses the partner typology developed by Martin, Vance, and Dean (1985) which facilitates the collection of partner type specific information for such variables as the total number of sexual partners or sexual occasions during the six months prior to the interview. Numbers of lifetime partners (separately for male and female sex partners) were established for 10-year periods and then summed up across these periods. The interview section on sexual practices covers only the past six months, and interviewees are asked how often they engaged in each practice in terms of the percent of the total times they had sex during this period. As a visual aid, the women in the study were presented with a "percent thermometer," with both descriptions of frequencies (e.g., all of the time, most of the time, etc.) and their number of sexual occasions marked beside the appropriate percent. The percentages were later converted by computer into absolute frequencies for each sexual practice.

Data Analysis

In analyzing the data, group comparison tests were used to examine differences between HIV+ and HIV− individuals. Both parametric and non-parametric statistical methods were applied, the latter because of frequent highly asymmetric distributions for numbers of sexual partners, numbers of sexual occasions, or numbers of different sexual practices. In examining sexual risk behaviors we did not use summary indices, but rather looked at individual behaviors in line with recent recommendations in the literature (Turner et al., 1989).

RESULTS

Sample Characteristics

As Table 1 shows, both groups of women (HIV+ and HIV−) are closely comparable in age, social status, levels of education, and income. The women tended to be in their thirties, many of them had not completed high school, and their income was low.

Approximately half of each of the two groups had never married, about 40% were divorced or separated, and only a minority of women (4 HIV+ and 5 HIV−) were currently married.

Most women were either Catholic or Protestant, with more Catholic women being HIV− (p = .06).

The majority of women in both groups were African-American, and the remainder divided about equally into Latina and Caucasian.

Female and Male Sex Partners

Sexual behavior was assessed for two time points, lifetime and past six months. One of the behavior categories assessed was indicators of homo/heterosexuality in regard to self-label and gender of sexual partner (see Table 2).

Although the majority of women were currently identified as heterosexuals, more women in the HIV+ group were self-identified as bisexual or lesbian (39.5%) than were women in the HIV− group (16.2%). This differ-

TABLE 1. Sample Characteristics by HIV Status (N = 75)[a]

Variables	HIV+ (N = 38)		HIV– (N = 37)		t-test p
	Mean	SD	Mean	SD	(2-tailed)
Age at interview (yrs.)	37.8	6.0	37.2	7.7	.68
Social status (Hollingshead 2F)	35.4	11.7	34.4	13.0	.84
Education (yrs. of school completed)	11.9	2.0	11.3	1.7	.15
Level of occupation (Hollingshead)	4.5	2.0	4.6	2.2	.85
Household income ($)	11,460	13,482	9,634	6,097	.46

Current marital status	N (38)	%	N (36)	%	Chi-Square p
Never married	19	50.0	17	47.2	
Married	4	10.5	5	13.9	.90
Divorced/separated	15	39.5	14	38.9	

Current religion	N (37)	%	N (37)	%	
Protestant	19	51.4	11	30.0	
Catholic	7	18.9	16	43.2	.06
Other	—	—	5	13.5	"Other"
No formal rel/None	11	29.7	5	13.5	and "No formal/ None" combined

Ethnicity	N (38)	%	N (37)	%	
White non-Hispanic	6	15.8	7	18.9	
Hispanic	4	10.5	9	24.3	.22
African-American	28	73.0	21	56.8	

[a] A few women with missing information were omitted from some of the analyses.

TABLE 2. Indicators of Homo/Heterosexuality in HIV+ and HIV– Women

Variables	HIV+		HIV–		Chi-Square p[a]
	N (38)	%	N (37)	%	
Sexual identity					
Self-label (current)					
Straight	22	57.9	31	83.8	
Bisexual	10	26.3	4	10.8	.04
Gay/Lesbian	5	13.2	2	5.4	(straight vs. non-
Other	1	2.6	—	—	straight)
Sexual partners, lifetime					
Had no partners, abstinent	—	—	—	—	
Had male partners only	17	44.7	22	59.5	.30
Had female partners only	—	—	—	—	
Had male and female partners	21	55.3	15	40.5	
Sexual partners, past 6 months					
Had no partners, abstinent	8	21.1	4	10.8	.37
Had male partners only	25	65.8	32	86.5	(no partner
Had female partners only	1	2.6	—	—	vs. all others
Had male and female partners	4	10.5	1	2.7	combined)

[a] With Yates correction.

ence in current self-labeling of sexual orientation was statistically significant (p = .04).

Current self-labeling as bisexual or lesbian did not correspond to either historical or current sexual activity with a same-sex partner. Fewer women self-identified as lesbian or bisexual than reported a history of bisexual behavior, and while significantly fewer HIV+ than HIV− women self-identified as straight or heterosexual, the proportion of women who reported having had female sex partners over their lifetime was comparable in both groups (55.3 among HIV+ vs. 40.5% among HIV− women). No women reported a history of female sex partners only.

The group difference in current self-labeling also did not entirely correspond to sexual behavior as indicated by gender of sex partners. Current sexual behavior (during the past six months) was mostly described by women in both groups as heterosexual (i.e., only 5 HIV+ women and one HIV− woman reported any sexual activity with a female partner). Of these five HIV+ women, three described women as their most frequent sexual partners (one of them had had no male partners and only one female partner); for a fourth woman, the sexual frequency with her most frequent (of 21) male sex partners was the same as with her one female partner; the fifth had a male as her most frequent sex partner. Additionally, one HIV− woman reported being sexually active with one man and two women, and identified her most frequent sex partner as a woman.

Lifetime Number of Sex Partners and Sex Occasions

The lifetime number of sex partners is an indicator of risk of HIV transmission, and the number of sex occasions represents sexual frequency.

Overall, the HIV+ women reported more male sex partners than did the HIV− women (Table 3), with medians of 26.5 vs. 11, which was statistically significant (p = .02). The range was large, with some women reporting as few as two or three and some as many as thousands of male sex partners, particularly if sex was exchanged for drugs and money (see following). HIV+ and HIV− women did not significantly differ in reported number of sex occasions.

Among those women who reported having had female sex partners, the number of female partners and sex occasions was much lower. HIV+ women tended to have had more female sex partners than HIV− women (medians 3 vs. 2), but did not differ in number of sexual occasions with women.

Overall, the HIV+ women had significantly more sex partners than HIV− women, as reflected in the combined numbers of male and female

TABLE 3. Lifetime Number of Sex Partners and Number of Sex Occasions

VARIABLE	HIV+					HIV−					
	N[a]	RANGE	MEDIAN	MEAN	SD	N[a]	RANGE	MEDIAN	MEAN	SD	MW[b] p
# of male partners	38	3-22,688	26.5	961.9	3705.6	37	2-52,709	11	2236.5	9668.3	.02
# of sex occasions with males	38	9-26,000	1749.5	3371.3	5488.0	36	4-112,300	2333.5	7129.1	19300.0	.26
# of female partners	21	1-55	3	8.6	13.2	15	1-14	2	2.7	3.3	.06
# of sex occasions with females	21	1-8,402	340	1592.8	2411.9	15	1-1,506	50	292.1	483.2	.22
# of male and female partners	38	3-22,688	32	966.6	3749.6	37	2-52,711	11	2237.6	9668.7	.005
# of male and female sexual occasions	38	148-26,000	2169	4251.5	5609.2	36	105-112,320	2556.5	7250.8	19333.6	.96

[a] A few women with missing information omitted.
[b] Mann-Whitney U test (2-tailed p, corrected for ties).

partners (p = .005). However, there were no significant differences between the groups in terms of estimates of total numbers of sexual occasions over their lifetime. Thus, HIV+ women had as much sexual activity as HIV − women, but changed partners more frequently.

Number of Male Sex Partners and Partner Risk Characteristics (Past Six Months)

Since for most women sexual behavior during the past six months involved only men, we will limit our discussion on number and risk characteristics to male partners only.

Most of the women in both groups had been sexually active with male partners in the six months prior to interview with the exception of nine HIV+ and four HIV − women who had had no male sex partner (Table 4). Many women in both groups were monogamous and had had sex with one man only (44.8% among HIV+ women and 66.7% among HIV − women). The majority of women reported having a male primary sex partner, the man with whom they had sex more than with anyone else during the past six months (82.8% vs. 100%), and 55.2% vs. 33.3% had additional partners with whom they had had sex on one or more occasions (data not shown). Overall, the two groups did not significantly differ in the number of male sex partners or occasions.

In addition to numbers of partners, the risk characteristics of male partners are important as an indication of sexual risk behavior for HIV transmission.

Overall, women often did not know important specifics about their male partners' risk history such as their HIV serostatus, history of blood transfusion, STDs, or bisexuality, but most women knew if their primary partner had had an injected drug history (see Table 5). About half of the women in each group did not know whether their primary partner was HIV − or HIV+; the others reported that their primary partners had been tested, and more primary partners of HIV+ women had tested as seropositive than did partners of HIV − women. Very few women reported blood transfusions or STDs, and none bisexuality among their primary partners. The women had very little knowledge about their other (than primary) male partners except for injected drug use which was known to six HIV+ women and two HIV − women.

Sex with Men for Money or Drugs (Past Six Months)

A subgroup of women in both groups engaged in sex with a male partner for money or drugs (see Table 6). Among the HIV+ women,

TABLE 4. Male Sex Partners of Women Who Were Sexually Active During the 6 Months Prior to Interview

Variable	HIV+		HIV−		Chi-Square[a]
	N	%	N	%	p
Abstinence from males	(N = 38)		(N = 37)		
Had no male sex partner	9	23.7	4	10.8	.24
Had 1 or more male sex partner	29	76.3	33	89.2	
Monogamy	(N = 29)		(N = 33)		
Was monogamous	13	44.8	22	66.7	.14
Had more than 1 male partner	16	55.2	11	33.3	

	(N = 29)				(N = 33)				MW[b]
	Range	Median	Mean	SD	Range	Median	Mean	SD	p
# of male partners	1-362	2	(22.8	78.9)	1-198	1	(9.1	34.6)	.13
# of sex occasions with males	1-560	20.0	(72.1	120.8)	1-360	48	(63.0	74.0)	.57

[a] With Yates correction.
[b] Mann-Whitney U test (2-tailed p, corrected for ties).

TABLE 5. Risk Characteristics of Male Partners of Women Who Were Sexually Active During the Past 6 Months Prior to Interview

Variable	HIV+		HIV−		Chi-Square[b]
	N	%	N	%	p
Primary male partner:	(N = 24)[a]		(N = 33)[a]		
AIDS/ARC/HIV+					
Negative test	5	20.8	13	39.4	NA
Not tested, DK	13	54.2	18	54.5	
Suspect positive	1	4.2	—	—	
Positive test	5	28.8	2	6.1	
Injected drug history (ever)					
Yes	17	70.8	21	63.6	.78
No or DK	7	29.2	12	36.4	
Blood transfusion, 1977-1985					
Yes	1	4.3	3	9.1	NA
No or DK	22	95.7	30	90.9	
STD in past 6 months					
Positive test	3	12.5	0	0	NA
Suspect positive	0	0	2	6.1	
No or DK	21	87.5	31	93.9	
Had sex with men					
No or DK	24	100	30	100[c]	NA
Other male partners:	(N = 17)		(N = 11)		
AIDS/ARC/HIV+, # of partners					
0 partners	17	100	10	90.9	NA
1 partner	0	0	1	9.1	

Injected drug history (ever)

# of partners

0 partners	11	64.7	9	81.8	NA
1 partner	6	35.3	1	9.1	
2 partners	0	—	1	9.1	

Blood transfusion, 1977-1985

# of partners

0 partners	17	100	11	100	NA

STD in past 6 months

# of partners

0 partners	17	100	11	100	NA

Other male partners had sex
  with men

# of partners

0 partners	17	100	10	90.9	NA
1 partner	0	—	1	9.1	

[a] Based on the number of women with the specified partner type. One HIV+ woman
   with missing information was omitted from Transfusion analysis.
[b] With Yates correction; NA = not applicable.
[c] Three women had missing information.

43.3%, and among the HIV − women, 27.3% reported having been paid for sex. For most women, this activity occurred with a limited number of partners, except for four HIV+ and three HIV − women who had received money for sex from 10 or more partners.

Only a small number of women (five HIV+ and four HIV −) reported engaging in sex with men for drugs.

Sexual Risk Behavior with Male and Female Partners
(Past Six Months)

Women were asked about the types of sexual behaviors in which they engaged, separately for male and female partners in the six months prior to interview. The interview included questions about non-genital activities (such as kissing and caressing); manual, oral, anal, and genital contact

TABLE 6. Sex for Money or Drugs in Women Who Were Sexually Active with Male Partners During the Six Months Prior to Interview

Variable	HIV+		HIV−		MW[b]
	N	%	N	%	p
	(N = 28)		(N = 33)		
# of partners: W was paid for sex					
0 partners	17	56.7	24	72.7	.22
1 partner	4	13.3	5	15.2	
2-4 partners	5	16.7	1	3.0	
10-30 partners	2	3.3	2	6.0	
197-360 partners	2	6.7	1	3.0	
# of occasions: W was paid for sex[a]					
1 occasion	2	16.7	1	11.1	.28
2-10 occasions	8	66.7	3	33.3	
30-49 occasions	0	0	4	44.4	
240-360 occasions	2	16.7	1	11.1	
# of partners: W received drugs for sex					
0 partners	24	82.8	29	87.9	.59
1 partner	2	6.9	2	6.1	
2-10 partners	3	10.3	2	6.1	
# of occasions: W received drugs for sex[a]					
1 occasion	1	20.0	2	50.0	.62
2-12 occasions	4	80.0	1	25.0	
50 occasions	0	—	1	25.0	

[a]% expressed of women (W) who were sexually active in the respective situation.
[b]Mann-Whitney U test (2-tailed p) for continuous data where applicable;
NA = not applicable.

with genitals; manual and oral contact with anus; and questions focused on transmission risk such as condom use, contact with ejaculate or vaginal fluids, contact with urine or feces, and practices that might draw blood.

There were no significant group differences in the percent of women who used a specific sexual practice. Vaginal intercourse was the most common sexual practice with men (see Table 7), and 55.2% vs. 42.4% (HIV+ vs. HIV −) reported using condoms at least once during intercourse. However, the majority of women also reported that their partners had ejaculated without condoms at least once into their vagina, indicating inconsistent condom use for a very high number of women in both groups.

Fellatio and cunnilingus were also practiced by most of the women in both groups and rarely with protection by condoms or any protective wrap.

Sexual practices in which less than a third of each group engaged included insertion of fingers into the rectum and oral/anal contact ("rimming"), both of which were more commonly practiced with the male partner as inserter and both of which were slightly more common among the HIV+ group. Anal intercourse was practiced by roughly 10% of the sample as a whole. Condoms were never used for this practice. Other sexual practices were extremely rare or not practiced at all by either group of women (e.g., urinating on partner's skin, contact with feces, etc.).

Among the small number of women who reported sexual behaviors with female sex partners over the last six months, the most common sexual practices were mutual masturbation and cunnilingus, ranging from three to 96 occasions in the six months. One HIV+ woman reported practices such as use of vaginal insertables on her partner, as well as "rimming," "fisting," and urination on her partner's skin. No form of HIV protection was used in any of these situations. Transmission risk through contact with blood was reported by one HIV+ woman and one HIV − woman, and this was related to sexual activity during menstruation. Overall, only one woman, from the HIV+ group, reported safer sex precautions during sexual activity with another woman (using glove or condom when inserting her finger in her partner's rectum).

Drug and Alcohol Use During Sex in the Six Months Prior to Interview

Drug and alcohol use during sex was extremely common; only one woman in each group reported no substance use during sex. In comparing the types of drugs used during sex by the HIV+ and HIV − groups, no statistically significant differences were found. However, the most common drugs used during sex among the HIV+ group were crack (smokable cocaine), methadone, and cocaine, whereas the most common drugs

TABLE 7. Percent of Women Engaging in a Given Sexual Practice, Among Participants Who Were Sexually Active with Male Partners in the Six Months Prior to Interview

Activity	HIV+ (N = 29) %	HIV− (N = 33) %	Chi-Square p
Vaginal intercourse	100	100	N.A.
with condom	55.2	42.4	.45
ejaculate into vagina, w/o condom (ever)	86.2	97.0	N.A.
Fellatio	72.4	69.7	1.00
with condom	17.2	6.1	N.A.
semen swallowed	20.7	27.3	.76
Cunnilingus	75.9	78.8	1.00
with wrap	0.0	3.0	N.A.
Masturbation of partner	71.4	66.7	.90
Masturbation by partner	60.7	66.7	.83
Ejaculate contact with skin	24.1	33.3	.60
Manual-anal fingering of partner	24.1	15.2	.57
with glove	—	3.0	N.A.
Manual-anal fingering by partner	27.6	18.2	.56
with glove	—	—	N.A.
Oral-anal "rimming"			
of partner	17.2	12.1	N.A.
by partner	27.6	15.2	.37
Anal intercourse	10.3	9.1	N.A.
with condom	—	—	N.A.
ejac. into rectum w/o condom	10.3	9.1	N.A.

among the HIV − group were methadone, alcohol, and cocaine. From a list of 14 drugs, only amyl nitrite ("poppers") was not used in either group.

The use of more than one substance in the six months prior to interview was also very common: the largest proportion of women in each group reported having used between one and three drugs; a sizeable proportion of both groups also reported having used between four and six drugs. Among the HIV+ women, 60% reported using between one and three drugs during sexual occasions (compared to 45.4% of the HIV − group); an additional 30% of the HIV+ women reported using between four and six drugs (compared to 32.4% of the HIV − group); an additional 6.7% of the HIV+ women reported using seven drugs (compared to 9.1% of the HIV − group reporting seven or eight drugs).

Pregnancy and Birth Control

Women not only have to consider protection from HIV and STDs when they engage in sexual behavior with a man, but also birth control against the risk of unwanted pregnancies. Of the 75 women participating in the study, 70 reported that they had not been pregnant during the past six months (see Table 8). Three women reported that they had become pregnant during that time; one miscarried and two had abortions. Two women provided no data with regard to pregnancy.

When the women participating in the study were asked about methods they or their partner used for birth control, the majority of the HIV+ women who had male sex partners reported that their partner used condoms for birth control (51.7%); however, data on sexual-risk practices indicate that condom use is sporadic and not consistent. Only 21.2% among the HIV − women reported condom use for birth control. The majority (57.6%) of women in the HIV − group reported no birth-control method at all.

Three women in each group reported that they had had tubal ligation to prevent pregnancies. A few women in each group reported use of the sponge, the rhythm method, or a combination of methods.

DISCUSSION

Our study describes the sexual behavior of women with a history of injected drug use and suggests that risk behavior for STD/HIV infection is common in this population. While our findings have limitations, since they are based on relatively small convenience samples, we have no reason to believe that the women participating in the study are not typical of patients of inner-city infectious disease clinics and methadone programs. Both groups of HIV+ and HIV − women were comparable in ethnicity, age, education, and social status. They only differed in religion, with more HIV+ women being Protestant and more HIV − women being Catholic.

TABLE 8. Pregnancy/Birth Control During the Past 6 Months Prior to Interview

Variable	HIV+		HIV–		Chi-Square
	N	%	N	%	p
Outcome of Pregnancy	(N = 38)[a]		(N = 37)[a]		
Miscarriage	1	2.6	0	—	
Artificial Termination	1	2.6	1	2.7	
Not Pregnant	35	92.2	35	94.6	
Birth	0	—	0	—	n.s.[b]
No Data	1	2.6	1	2.7	
Birth Control Used [b]	(N = 28)[a]		(N = 33)[a]		
None	11	37.9	19	57.6	
Pill	0	—	0	—	
Injectible	0	—	0	—	
IUD	0	—	0	—	
Spermicide	0	—	0	—	
Diaphragm	0	—	0	—	.041[c]
Tubal Ligation	3	10.3	3	9.1	
Sponge	0	—	1	3.0	
Rhythm Method	0	—	1	3.0	
Male Uses Condom	15	51.7	7	21.2	
Male Uses Withdrawal	0	—	0	—	
Multiple	0	—	2	6.1	

[a] N reflects all sexually active subjects
[b] Pregnant vs. not pregnant, by HIV status: n.s.
[c] 3 × 2 table: (A) None vs. (B) Male Uses Condom vs. (C) Other/Multiple Birth Control Methods, by HIV status. Individual 2 × 2 tables: (A) vs. (B + C) n.s. (Chi-square p = 0.12); (B) vs. (C) p = 0.06 (Fisher's Exact Test, 2-tailed).

Whether religious identification was a factor in explaining some of the differences in behavior between the two groups is difficult to ascertain.

Overall, both groups tended to be more similar than different in their current sexual behavior, suggesting that the knowledge of positive HIV status has a limited effect, if any, on behavior in this population.

One of the surprising findings of our study is related to sexual orientation and self-identification as heterosexual, bisexual, or lesbian. A substantial number of women in both groups did not identify as heterosexual but as bisexual or lesbian; this was significantly more so among the HIV+ women.

Although HIV − women were not different in their lifetime bisexual behavior from HIV+ women, fewer HIV − women labeled themselves as bisexual or lesbian. This finding is puzzling and requires an explanation that is not readily apparent. We currently lack population norms on lifetime bisexual behavior among women, especially among African-Americans and Latinas. Thus, it is impossible to determine whether such bisexual behavior is typical among women with similar social demographics or whether it is a characteristic of injected drug using women. Ross et al. (1992) reported a similar finding in a Sydney sample of injected drug users in regard to the high prevalence of self-identified and behavioral lesbianism and the high prevalence of HIV+ lesbians. Usually, bisexual behavior and bisexual self-label are not assessed as part of sexual risk behavior in women and are hardly ever addressed in prevention programs. Our results suggest that this is an omission that requires change. Since self-identification as straight, bisexual, or gay does not necessarily indicate exclusive behavior with one type of sex partner, education and prevention for all women need to be comprehensive. In particular, women who identify as gay or lesbian have been excluded from educational and prevention programs because of the erroneous assumption that the self-label signifies exclusive sexual behavior with female partners, a behavior which is deemed of low risk for HIV infection. Our findings agree with others who report that many lesbian women also engage in sexual behavior with men (Blumstein and Schwartz, 1983; Reinisch, Sanders, and Ziemba-Davis, 1988) and therefore are at risk for STD/HIV infection.

While HIV+ and HIV − women differed in numbers of lifetime male and female sexual partners, their current sexual behavior was not different in this respect. The greater number of lifetime partners among HIV+ women may have been a factor in their becoming infected with HIV, although sexual risk behavior and needle sharing obviously put this group of women in double jeopardy.

Current sexual behavior revealed abstinence among a small number of women, monogamy for half to two-thirds of women, and many male partners for a small number of women, sometimes in exchange for money and, rarely, in exchange for drugs. In none of these behaviors did the two groups differ from each other, and there was little evidence that knowledge of HIV positivity had a strong effect on partner frequency.

The majority of women in both groups knew that their male partner had been an injected drug user, but only a few knew their partner's HIV status, STD history, or possible bisexual behavior. This lack of information was even more pronounced for more casual partners outside of the primary sex partner. We did not collect information on whether the women in our study had attempted to find out about their partners' sexual risk behavior. Even if they had done so, however, taking one's partner's sexual risk history is not an effective practice and has been shown to be of dubious value as an HIV-prevention strategy (Mays and Cochran, 1988).

The most alarming finding of our study is the frequency of unprotected sexual practices among both HIV+ and HIV − women, with 86% of HIV+ and 97% of HIV − women reporting inconsistent or no condom use for vaginal intercourse, thus clearly risking HIV infection for themselves and their sex partners. This sample of women is not too different from other groups of women and men in the U.S., since there is little evidence that consistent condom use has become routine among heterosexuals (Ehrhardt, Yingling, and Warne, 1991).

In interpreting our results, it is important to emphasize that condom use is often not under a woman's control since it requires the male partner's cooperation. Thus, there is an urgent public health need to develop new methods that can be controlled by women, such as the female condom or a virucide (Stein, 1990).

Another important finding was the common use of drugs and alcohol during sex, clearly an additional disinhibitor against taking precautions. Thus, any effective prevention program needs to tackle strategies for insuring safer sex as well as for treatment of substance use beyond injected drug use.

Finally, contraceptive behavior for birth control as reported by the women in our study was not very effective and requires attention.

In summary, we conclude that sexual risk behavior among inner-city women with a history of injected drug use needs to be assessed in detail in order to form the basis for appropriate educational efforts and more effective behavior change programs.

AUTHOR NOTE

This work was supported in part by Center Grant 5-P50-MH43520 from NIMH and NIDA to the first author. Eden Kainer, Jennifer Hay, Gregg Gottehrer, and Ramani Durvasula served as research assistants.

REFERENCES

Battjes, R., & Pickens, R. (1988). *AIDS transmission among IVDUs.* IV International Conference on AIDS (Abstract No. 8008), Stockholm, Sweden.

Blumstein, P.W., & Schwartz, P. (1983). *American couples: Money, work, and sex.* New York: Morrow.

Centers for Disease Control. (1992). *HIV/AIDS surveillance report, March.*

Ehrhardt, A.A., Yingling, S., & Warne, P. (1991). Sexual behavior in the era of AIDS: What has changed in the United States? *Annual Review of Sex Research 2,* 25-47.

Gruen, R.S., & Meyer-Bahlburg, H.F.L. (1992). *Training manual for research interviews about sexual behavior.* Unpublished manuscript, Columbia University, Department of Psychiatry, New York City.

Harris, R., Langrod, J., & Hebert, J. (1990). Changes in AIDS risk behavior among intravenous drug abusers in New York City. *New York State Journal of Medicine 4,* March, 123-126.

Martin, J.L., Vance, C.S. & Dean, L.L. (1985). *The impact of AIDS on healthy gay men: A research instrument.* Unpublished manuscript, Columbia University, Division of Sociomedical Sciences, School of Public Health, New York City.

Mays, V.M. & Cochran, S.D. (1988). Issues in the perception of AIDS risk and risk reduction activities by Black and Hispanic/Latina women. *American Psychologist, 43*(11), 949-957.

Meyer-Bahlburg, H.F.L., & Ehrhardt, A.A. (1983). *Sexual behavior assessment schedule–Adult* (SEBAS-A). Unpublished manuscript, Columbia University, Department of Psychiatry, New York City.

Meyer-Bahlburg, H.F.L., Ehrhardt, A.A., Exner, T.M., Calderwood, M., & Gruen, R.S. (1988). *Sexual risk behavior assessment schedule–Adult, baseline interview for female drug users* (SERBAS-A-DF-1). Unpublished manuscript, Columbia University, Department of Psychiatry, New York City.

Meyer-Bahlburg, H.F.L., Exner, T., Lorenz, G., Gruen, R.S., & Gorman, J.M. (1991). Sexual risk behavior, sexual functioning and HIV-disease progression in gay men. *Journal of Sex Research, 28*(1), 3-27.

Reinisch, J.M., Sanders, S.A., & Ziemba-Davis, M. (1988). The study of sexual behavior in relation to the transmission of HIV. *American Psychologist, 43,* 921-927.

Ross, M.W., Wodak, A., Gold, J., & Miller, M.E. (1992). Differences across sexual orientation on HIV risk behaviours in injecting drug users. *AIDS Care, 4,* 139-148.

Stein, Z. (1990). HIV prevention: The need for methods women can use. *American Journal of Public Health, 80,* 460-462.

Turner, C.F., Miller, H.G., & Moses, L.E. (1989). *AIDS: Sexual behavior and intravenous drug use.* Washington, D.C.: National Academy Press.

Stages of Sexual Behavior Change to Reduce the Risk of HIV/AIDS: The Chicago MACS/CCS Cohort

S. Maurice Adib, MD, DrPH
David G. Ostrow, MD, PhD

SUMMARY. Sexual behavior change to reduce the risk of HIV infection is a dynamic multi-staged process. We present an empirical model for change, where we describe a stage of initiation of safer sexual practices, followed by a consolidation stage, and a long-term maintenance stage. The process of change can be interrupted by occasional or repeated lapses. We apply this multi-stage model to sexual behavior in a cohort of gay men from the Chicago area. The prevalence of various stages are reported between 1986 and 1991. Men infected with HIV tended to initiate change to safer sex later than those who were not, but maintained change or relapsed to unsafe practices in the same proportion. Implications regarding factors associated with relapse to unsafe sex, and interventions to prevent relapse, are discussed. *[Single or multiple copies of this article are available from The Haworth Document Delivery Service: 1-800-342-9678, 9:00 a.m. - 5:00 p.m. (EST).]*

S. Maurice Adib is affiliated with the University of Michigan, School of Public Health, Ann Arbor, MI. David G. Ostrow is also affiliated with the University of Michigan, School of Public Health, Ann Arbor, MI, and the Medical College of Wisconsin, Community Behavior Program, Milwaukee, WI.

[Haworth co-indexing entry note]: "Stages of Sexual Behavior Change to Reduce the Risk of HIV/AIDS: The Chicago MACS/CCS Cohort." Adib, S. Maurice, and David G. Ostrow. Co-published simultaneously in *Journal of Psychology & Human Sexuality* (The Haworth Press, Inc.) Vol. 7, No. 1/2, 1995, pp. 121-133; and: *HIV/AIDS and Sexuality* (ed: Michael W. Ross) The Haworth Press, Inc., 1995, pp. 121-133; and: *HIV/AIDS and Sexuality* (ed: Michael W. Ross) Harrington Park Press, an imprint of The Haworth Press, Inc., 1995, pp. 121-133. *[Single or multiple copies of this article are available from The Haworth Document Delivery Service: 1-800-342-9678, 9:00 a.m. - 5:00 p.m. (EST).]*

121

INTRODUCTION

Many behavioral scientists regard sexual change to reduce HIV risk as a multi-staged process, but they generally differ in the definition of the number of stages, and the significance of each stage in the process (Catania, Kegeles, Coates, 1990; O'Reilly, Higgins, Galavotti, Sheridan, 1990). A variety of articles dealing with behavioral change among men who have sex with men have focused on one stage of change, such as initiation and maintenance of safer sexual practices, or lapse to unsafe practices (Ekstrand & Coates, 1990; de Wit, van Griensven, Kok, Sandfort, 1993; Ekstrand, 1992; Stall, Ekstrand, Pollack, McKusick, Coates, 1990). These articles, as well as a series of analyses reported over time from a cohort of gay men in Chicago (Adib, Joseph, Ostrow, Tal, Schwartz, 1991; Emmons et al., 1986; Joseph et al., 1987) demonstrate clearly that the significance of psychosocial factors affecting HIV-related sexual behavior vary with each stage of change (Catania et al., 1990; Peterson, Ostrow, McKirnan, 1991). These stages therefore correspond to the realities of different persons engaging in similar types of sexual behavior but at different periods during a long-term process of change. Thus, we can differentiate, for example, between engaging in unsafe practices while initiating change, and engaging in those same practices after a period of change towards safer behavior. The latter event is considered a 'lapse.' 'Lapsing' per se is conceived as an isolated occurrence of unsafe sexual practice, usually under the effect of transient circumstances, such as intoxication, emotional status, or unavailability of condoms. We use the concept of 'relapse' when a repetitive pattern of lapsing is observed. The recurrence of lapses, or relapse, is believed to indicate a concomitant change in an individual's more permanent characteristics, such as coping strategies, social environment, personal attitudes, psychological predisposition, and relationship status (Marlatt and Gordon, 1980).

In this paper, we have described the stages of HIV sexual behavior change among gay men in Chicago participating simultaneously in the Chicago Multicenter AIDS Cohort Study (MACS) and the Coping and Change Study (CCS). At various periods during a five year follow-up period (1986-1991), participants entered stages of initiation, consolidation, and maintenance of change to safer receptive anal sex (RAS) practices, and possibly lapsed or relapsed (Figure 1). We report the prevalence of these stages over time.

For the purposes of this paper, safer practices included either consistent condom use when engaging in RAS or avoidance of this specific practice altogether, while unsafe sex meant any episode of unprotected RAS. This definition of 'unsafe sex' can be disputed, since the nature of the relationship between sexual partners and their HIV serostatus, may render some episodes of unprotected anal sex less 'unsafe' than others (Hart, Boulton, Fitzpatrick, McLean, Dawson, 1992). However, it has been argued that such mitigating elements cannot be assessed in an accurate manner, by the individuals engaging in sex nor by objective observers, and therefore it is necessary to consider all unprotected episodes as potentially risky events that should be avoided or prevented (Ekstrand et al., 1993). The definition adopted in this paper is not intended to defend or oppose such behavioral arguments. The CCS dataset available for this analysis simply does not include the dyadic information necessary for the distinction between various types of unprotected anal sex episodes. Nevertheless, findings stemming from this analysis remain important from an epidemiological point of view, in assessing the potential for acquiring/transmitting HIV among cohorts of urban gay men.

METHODS

Cross-Sectional Behavioral Outcomes

Data were collected from self-identified gay men participating since 1984 in the Chicago component of the Multicenter AIDS Cohort Study (MACS). These men were concurrently recruited into a semi-annual psychosocial and behavioral Coping and Change Study (CCS). The sampling of the cohort and the study design have been described in previous publications (Emmons et al., 1986; Kaslow et al., 1987). In particular, the CCS questionnaire elicited data regarding lifetime and prior month practice of receptive anal sex (RAS), a practice entailing the highest risk for HIV infection among men who have sex with men (Kingsley et al., 1987).

Starting January 1986, at visit 4 (V4) of the Chicago MACS/CCS, detailed information regarding condom use in the previous month were added to the RAS section of the questionnaire. Based on their responses on that section, participants were classified, from V4 on, into one of two cross-sectional categories (Adib et al., 1991):

1. *Safer RAS practices:* avoidance of RAS, or consistent condom use.
2. *Unsafe RAS practices:* inconsistent or no condom use during RAS.

Definition of Longitudinal Panel Participants Analysis

A longitudinal panel of V4 participants was defined as those men who had completed at least two out of every three visits between V4 and V15

(June 1991). Of the 672 participants at V4, 396 (59%) fulfilled the panel definition.

The Empirical Model of Stages of Behavioral Change to Reduce Risk of HIV Infection

An empirical model was defined to include various stages experienced by participants as they proceed to change their sexual behavior to reduce the risk of HIV infection. Basically, the change process consists of a 3-stage hierarchical sequence. Each stage combined reports from three consecutive visits (Figure 1):

1. *Initiation of change:* inconsistent practice of safer sex among men reporting prior unsafe RAS behavior. In this stage, safer practices are reported for the first time either at one or two intervening visits.
2. *Consolidation of change:* consistent practice of safer sex following initiation of change. In this stage, safer practices are reported for the first time at all three intervening visits.
3. *Maintenance of change:* consistent practice of safer sex following consolidation of change. In this stage, safer practices continue to be reported at all three intervening visits. This stage is the safest final stage of behavior change identified in this study.

The model assumes that consolidation of change always follows initiation. However, some participants who had been engaging in unsafe sex attained a consolidation stage without going through an *observable* initiation stage due to the limited one-month recall period. Therefore, participants who entered the consolidation stage after a brief period of inconsistently safe behavior outside of the retrospective recall period may not be identified.

Along the 3-stage hierarchical sequence from initiation to maintenance of change, lapse to unsafe sex can occur. A lapse is defined as at least one instance of unsafe sexual practices following any one of the above three stages. An individual can recover from a first lapse stage and re-enter the change sequence through a consolidation stage. When a lapse occurs again, the individual enters a *relapse* stage. The follow-up period between 1986 and 1991 was divided into 4 three-visit sub-periods (SP). During any given SP, participants could be found in any relevant stage of behavioral change, or in none (*'non-initiation'*).

The viability of this multi-stage model of RAS behavior change was tested directly by calculating the prospective risk of HIV infection among the initially seronegative participants in the MACS/CCS. The model pre-

FIGURE 1. Stages of Behavioral Change to Reduce Sexual Risk for HIV Infection

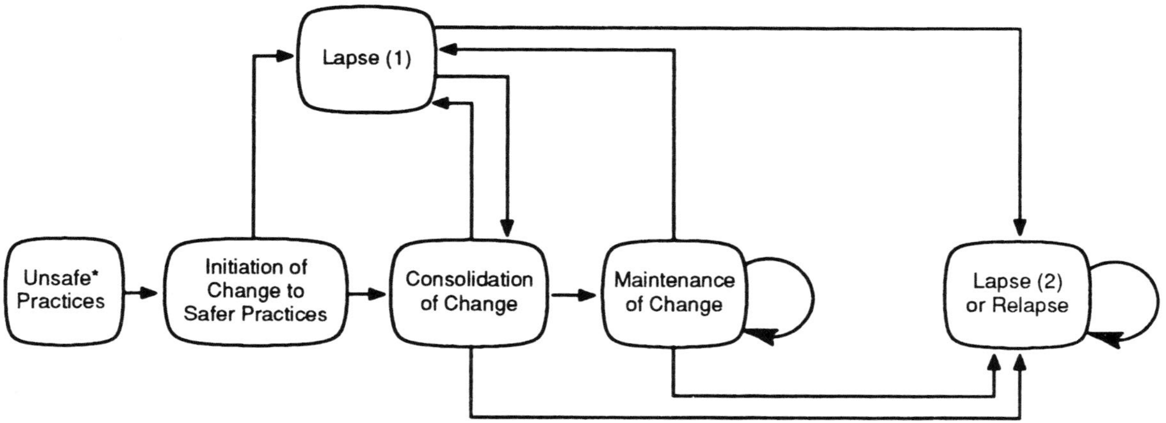

* Unsafe practices include engaging in receptive anal sex with inconsistent or no condom use, while safer practices include consistent condom use or avoidance of receptive anal sex.

dicts decreasing risk of HIV infection as men go through each stage of behavior change form initiation to consolidation, with increasing risk of infection occurring in the lapse/cumulative relapse conditions. As shown in Table 1, the rates of newly acquired HIV infection (as determined by the MACS using standardized testing procedures (Kaslow et al., 1987) for men observed in each stage were entirely in accord with the models predictions.

RESULTS

Description of the Panel

Panel participants were 396 homosexual men, mainly white (96%), 37 years old on average, with 16 years of educational attainment, and $21,000 of average annual income (in 1984-85). V4 participants who were not included in the panel did not differ from panelists on race, education, income, likelihood of seroconverting, or practice of RAS. Non-panelists were slightly younger (35 years old on average, p-value < 0.01), and more than twice as likely to be seropositive than panelists (Odds-ratio 2.4; 95% CI = 1-3.8). All but four participants reported engaging in RAS at some point prior to V4.

Stages of Sexual Behavior Change

In June 1986, at V4, 35% of panel participants reported engaging in mostly unsafe RAS in the previous month. The rest of the panel (65%) reported safer practices, mainly by not engaging in RAS. At subsequent visits, the proportion of men reporting safer practices increased steadily, to reach 90% by V12 (Figure 2).

Stages of sexual behavioral change were assessed by three-visit intervals between V4 and V15, based on the cross-sectional prevalence of RAS practices reported at each visit. Figure 3 presents the prevalence of these stages during the four sub-periods (SP) of follow-up. A cumulative analysis of behavioral stages of change indicated that all but 1% of panel participants entered an initiation stage at some point during the follow-up period.

Of those participants who initiated change to safer practices, 81% entered a consolidation stage at least once, and 76% entered a mainte- nance stage at least once. At any given SP, some participants lapsed, and subsequently either consolidated change to safer practices or relapsed.

TABLE 1. Seroconversion Rates by Stages of Sexual Behavior Change in the Chicago MACS/CCS Cohort (1986-1990)

Stages of Behavior Change	Number of Seroconverters/At-Risk Seronegative Men					Seroconversion rate/100 person years
	1986	1987	1988	1989	1990	
Non-Initiation (Consistently unsafe)	2/60	0/31	1/23	1/18	2/17	2.50
Initiation of Change	1/60	0/15	0/7	0/5	1/5	2.17
Lapse	NA	1/58	0/39	1/38	4/28	1.86
Relapse	NA	NA	0/38	3/65	11/93	1.64
Maintenance of Change	NA	1/135	2/132	2/136	8/135	0.89
Total Seroconverters	3/301	3/276	3/273	7/298	27/294	1.38

FIGURE 2. Cross-Sectional Prevalence of Safer Sexual Practices: Panel 1986-91 (N = 396)

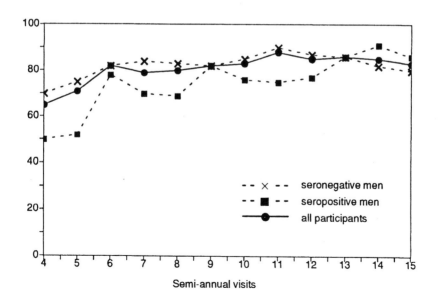

FIGURE 3. Prevalence of Stages of Behavioral Change to Reduce Risk for HIV Infection: RAS Panel 1986–1991 (N = 574)

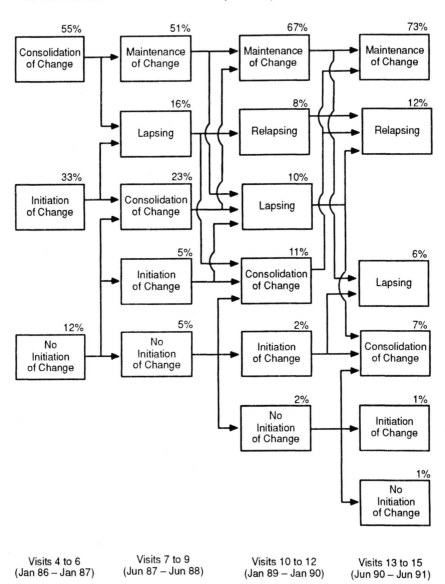

Visits 4 to 6
(Jan 86 – Jan 87)

Visits 7 to 9
(Jun 87 – Jun 88)

Visits 10 to 12
(Jan 89 – Jan 90)

Visits 13 to 15
(Jun 90 – Jun 91)

Table 2 presents the proportions of consolidation following lapse. Although large proportions of lapsers eventually consolidated safer practices (55% at SP3 and 63% at SP4), many did not but rather moved on into a relapse stage (45% at SP3 and 37% at SP4). Overall, 12% of the men had entered a relapse stage at the end of the five-year follow-up period.

Effect of HIV Serostatus on Stages of Behavioral Change

The prevalence of HIV infection in this panel was 27%, and 30 incident cases occurred during follow-up (7%). Cross-sectionally, HIV seropositive men were significantly more likely to report unsafe RAS at V4 than seronegative men. This difference decreased over time, and lost all significance after V8 (Figure 2).

At SP1, HIV seronegative men were more likely to have initiated safer RAS practices earlier than seropositive men (OR = 2.20; 95% CI: 2.03-2.37). Seropositive men were more likely to relapse than seronegative men, but the difference, although important, was not statistically significant (Figure 4). No other differences were found in the likelihood of consolidating or maintaining safer sex between the two serological subgroups.

DISCUSSION

This report describes a dynamic multi-stage process of sexual behavior change to reduce the risk of HIV infection from the practice of receptive

TABLE 2. Consolidation of Change to Safer Sexual Practices Following Lapse: Panel 1986-91 (N = 396)

	SP1 1/86-1/87	SP2 6/87-6/88	SP3 1/89-1/90	SP4 6/90-6/91
Lapse (% of panel participants)	NA	16%	10%	6%
Consolidation (% of those lapsing at the previous SP)	NA	NA	55%	63%
Relapse (%)	NA	NA	45%	37%

NA = Not Applicable

FIGURE 4. Stages of Behavioral Change by HIV Serostatus

(June 90 – June 91) (N = 396 MEN)

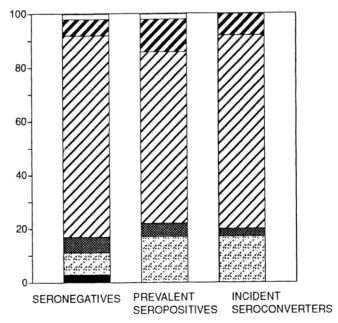

anal sex (RAS) among gay men in the Chicago MACS/CCS cohort. The change process has been empirically modeled over twelve semi-annual visits covering a five-year follow-up period (1986-91). The change process starts with a stage of initiation of safer practices, followed by a consolidation stage, then a maintenance stage. Reports of unsafe practices subsequent to entering any one of these three stages define a 'lapsing' stage. 'Lapsers' could return to a consolidation stage. Prospectively observed HIV infection rates among the initially uninfected men in the cohort lend substantial validity to this model.

All except a handful of participants had initiated some safer practices at various times during the 5-year follow-up period. At the end of the follow-up, a large proportion of participants (73%) were still in a maintenance stage, while 12% had lapsed repeatedly or 'relapsed.' HIV serostatus seemed to affect the change process only in the earliest period. Seropositive men were initially more likely to engage in unsafe practices, and tended to initiate change to safer sex later than seronegative men. No differences were to be found between the two serological groups at later periods.

Findings confirmed that initial isolated 'lapses' are likely to determine a more permanent 'relapse' status (Gold, Skinner, Grant, Plummer, 1991). Behavioral change to safer sex involves avoiding pleasurable practices previously engaged in, through a significant volitional effort. An initial return to the undesirable behavior (lapse) is associated with feelings of ineffectiveness in controlling sexual behavior, psychological distress, remorse, feelings of guilt and depression (Joseph et al., 1990; Hays, Turner, Coates, 1992). Such feelings can be expected to strongly undermine resolves to avoid further unsafe encounters, thus reducing self-efficacy, an important contributor to long-term maintenance of safer practices. It is therefore prudent to target interventions at preventing these initial lapses and/or preventing them from leading to a more permanent relapse pattern.

It can be argued epistemologically, that negotiated episodes of unsafe sex, agreed upon in advance after an informed assessment of risk involved with a specific HIV seroconcordant partner, are not actual lapses (Kippax, Crawford, Davis, Rodden, Dowsett, 1993). The Chicago MACS/CCS, like most longitudinal studies of sexual behavior, is limited in its ability to describe the dyadic context in which sex is performed. No data are available regarding the consistency of sexual partners and/or of their serostatus. Given these limitations, it is impossible for us to assess the prevalence of such negotiated lapses versus unexpected lapses. To successfully separate these two types of lapses, it would be necessary to use qualitative methods, such as interviews and diary analysis to complement data available through longitudinal studies.

Whatever the reasons behind a return to unprotected receptive anal sex, it is clear from this study that the resulting increased risk of HIV infection is significant, placing men at nearly the same rate of HIV infection as they were before initiating safer sex practices. Hopefully, this information, along with the availability of effective relapse prevention programs, can reduce the rate of new HIV infections among gay/bisexual men.

AUTHOR NOTE

This study was supported by a grant from NIMH to the Coping and Change Study (2RO1MH39346 and 1KO1MH00507). It was made possible by the Chicago Multicenter AIDS Cohort Study, funded by NIAID (AI32535), and the collaboration of the MACS Investigators John Phair, MD, and Joan Chmiel, PhD We greatly appreciate the constructive comments from our CCS collaborators Jill Joseph, PhD, and the practical support of Mrs. Bonnie Andree. We are also indebted to staff members of the Howard Brown Health Center in Chicago, and the participants who steadfastly provide the detailed intimate information which is the basis of this report. Findings have been partially reported at the VIIIth International Conference on AIDS, Amsterdam, 1992.

BIBLIOGRAPHY

Adib, S.M., Joseph, J.G., Ostrow, D.G., Tal, M., Schwartz, S.A. (1991). Relapse in sexual behavior among homosexual men: A 2-year follow-up from the Chicago MACS/CCS. *AIDS, 5*, 757-760.

Catania, J.A., Kegeles, S.M., Coates, T.J. (1990). Towards an understanding of risk behavior: An AIDS Risk Reduction Model (ARRM). *Health Educ Q, 17*, 53-72.

Ekstrand, M., Stall, R., Kegeles, S., Hays, R., DeMayo, M., Coates, T. (1993). Safer sex among gay men: What is the ultimate goal? *AIDS, 7*, 281-282.

Ekstrand, M.L. (1992). Safer sex maintenance among gay men: are we making any progress? *AIDS, 6*, 875-877.

Ekstrand, M.L. and Coates, T.J. (1990). Maintenance of safer sexual behaviors and predictors of risky sex: The San Francisco Men's Health Study. *Am J Public Health, 80*, 973-977.

Emmons, C.A., Joseph, J.G., Kessler, R.C., Wortman, C.B., Montgomery, S.B., Ostrow, D.G. (1986). Psychosocial predictors of reported behavior change in homosexual men at risk for AIDS. *Health Educ Q, 13*, 331-345.

Gold, R., Skinner, M., Grant, P., Plummer, D. (1991). Situational factors and thought processes associated with unprotected intercourse in gay men. *Psychol and Health, 5*, 259-278.

Hart, G., Boulton, M., Fitzpatrick, R., McLean, J., Dawson, J. (1992). 'Relapse' to unsafe sexual behaviour among gay men: A critique of recent behavioural HIV/AIDS research. *Sociology of Health and Illness, 14*, 216-232.

Hays, R.B., Turner, H., Coates, T.J. (1992). Social support, AIDS-related symptoms and depression among gay men. *J Consult Clinical Psychol, 60*, 463-469.

Joseph, J.G., Caumartin, S.M., Tal, M., Kirscht, J.P., Kessler, R., Ostrow, D.G., Wortman, C.B. (1990). Psychological functioning in a cohort of gay men at risk for AIDS. A three-year descriptive study. *J. Nervous Mental Diseases, 178*, 607-615.

Joseph, J.G., Montgomery, S.B., Emmons, C.A., Kessler, R.C., Ostrow, D.G., Wortman, C.B., O'Brien, K., Eller, M., and Eshleman, S. (1987). Magnitude and determinants of behavioral risk reduction: Longitudinal analysis of a cohort at risk for AIDS. *Psychol and Health, 1,* 73-96.

Kaslow, R.A., Ostrow, D.G., Detels, R., Phair, J.P., Polk, B.F., Rinaldo, C.R., Jr. (1987). The Multicenter AIDS Cohort Study: Rationale, organization and selected characteristics of the participants. *Am J Epidemiol, 126,* 310-318.

Kingsley, L.A., Kaslow, R., Rinaldo, C.R., Chmiel, J., Detre, K., Kelsey, S.F., Odaka, N., Ostrow D. et al. (1987). Risk factors for seroconversion to human immunodeficiency virus among male homosexuals. *Lancet 1,* 345-349.

Kippax, S., Crawford, J., Davis, M., Rodden, P., Dowsett, G. (1993). Sustaining safe sex: A longitudinal study of a sample of homosexual men. *AIDS, 7,* 257-263.

Marlatt, G.A. and Gordon, J.R. (1980). Determinants of relapse: Implications for the maintenance of behavioral change. In Davidson, P.O. and Davidson S.M. (Eds.), *Behavioral Medicine: Changing Health Lifestyles.* New York: Brunner/Mazel.

O'Reilly, K.R., Higgins, D.L., Galavotti, C., Sheridan, J. (1990). Relapse from safer sex among homosexual men: Evidence from four cohorts in the AIDS community demonstration projects. Proc VI International Conference on AIDS, San Francisco, (Abs. FC 717).

Peterson, P.L., Ostrow, D.G., and McKirnan, D.J. (1991). Behavioral interventions for primary prevention of HIV infection among homosexual/bisexual men. *J of Primary Prevention, 12,* 19-34.

Stall, R., Ekstrand, M., Pollack, L., McKusick, L., Coates, T. (1990). Relapse from safer sex: The next challenge for AIDS prevention efforts. *J Acquir Immune Defic Syndr, 3,* 1181-1187.

de Wit, J.B.F., van Griensven, G.J.P., Kok, G., Sandfort, T.G.M. (1993). Why do homosexual men relapse into unsafe sex? Predictors of resumption of unprotected anogenital intercourse with casual partners. *AIDS, 7,* 1113-1118.

Associations Among Coping Style, Personality, Unsafe Sexual Behavior, Depression, Conflict over Sexual Orientation, and Gender Nonconformity: HIV Status as a Modulating Variable

James D. Weinrich, PhD
J. Hampton Atkinson, MD
Thomas L. Patterson, PhD
J. Allen McCutchan, MD
John C. Gonsiorek, PhD
Igor Grant, MD
The HNRC Group

SUMMARY. Little attention has been given to dispositional variables in relapse into unsafe sex. In two previous papers, we showed (1) that recurrent adult depression in the gay/bisexual men in our

---

James D. Weinrich, J. Hampton Atkinson, Thomas L. Patterson, and J. Allen McCutchan, Igor Grant and the HNRC Group[1] are all affiliated with the University of California, San Diego. John C. Gonsiorek is affiliated with the University of Minnesota.

Address correspondence to James D. Weinrich, PhD, 2760 Fifth Avenue #200, San Diego, CA 92103.

[Haworth co-indexing entry note]: "Associations Among Coping Style, Personality, Unsafe Sexual Behavior, Depression, Conflict over Sexual Orientation, and Gender Nonconformity: HIV Status as a Modulating Variable." Weinrich, James D. et al. Co-published simultaneously in *Journal of Psychology & Human Sexuality* (The Haworth Press, Inc.) Vol. 7, No. 1/2, 1995, pp. 135-160; and: *HIV/AIDS and Sexuality* (ed: Michael W. Ross) The Haworth Press, Inc., 1995, pp. 135-160; and: *HIV/AIDS and Sexuality* (ed: Michael W. Ross) Harrington Park Press, an imprint of The Haworth Press, Inc., 1995, pp. 135-160. [Single or multiple copies of this article are available from The Haworth Document Delivery Service: 1-800-342-9678, 9:00 a.m. - 5:00 p.m. (EST).]

sample is often associated with high gender nonconformity, especially core gender dysphoria, in childhood, (2) that coping strategies
and personality scores are associated with changes from 1979 to
1989 in unsafe sex–defined as receiving semen rectally without a
condom (RSR), and (3) that sexual identity conflicts are related to a
general style of escape-avoidant coping, (4) which is in turn
associated with the MMPI profiles previously shown to correlate
with unsafe sex. Here we break down these analyses to see if these
patterns are related to HIV status.

We studied over 500 gay/bisexual men who contributed SCID
interviews, Freund Feminine Gender Identity scale scores, MMPI-2
profiles, Ways of Coping (Revised) scores, Profile of Mood States
(POMS) scores, and sex histories (*ns* varied by analysis).

Concerning the relationship between FGI and depression (1), we
found that the correlations persisted in the HIV positive subsample,
but vanished to insignificance among the HIV negative controls. A
similar pattern emerged in the correlations pertaining to MMPI scores
and unsafe sex (2), as well as in the association between escape-avoidant coping and sexual identity conflict (3). The analyses correlating
the MMPI scores with escape-avoidant coping were, in contrast,
equally strongly associated when broken down by HIV status.

A series of sample selection biases could account for these results.
It would be more parsimonious, however, to hypothesize a deeper
rationale. We suggest more investigation of the possibility that psychological and sexological variables may have more intriguing effects on sexual behaviors or the dispositional factors (perhaps even
immunologic ones) leading to HIV exposure than has been recog-
nized to date. *[Single or multiple copies of this article are available
from The Haworth Document Delivery Service: 1-800-342-9678,
9:00 a.m. - 5:00 p.m. (EST).]*

INTRODUCTION

It is remarkable how little attention has been given to understanding, at
the intrapsychic level, why people prefer some sexual activities over others. Although many sex researchers (turned AIDS researchers) and AIDS
researchers (turned sexologists) have discovered a great deal about sex
and AIDS, each discipline seems to have its own reasons for so little
investigating these deeper causes of the erotic preferences they wish
people to change or control in the face of the epidemic. Even disciplines
which might be naturally expected to investigate such questions (psychiatry and psychology), while showing much interest in population rates and
treatment strategies, have rarely explored the deeper relationships between

depression, personality, and unsafe sex. For example, a recent series of computer searches turned up only one paper on MMPI scores in a homosexual population (with an *n* of 35: Pakesch, Pfersmann, Loimer, Grunberger, Linzmayer, & Mayerhofer, 1992), and a mere handful on personality and safer sex (Clement, 1992; Kelly, St. Lawrence, & Brasfield, 1990; McCown, 1991, 1993; Ross, 1986, 1988, 1990)–if personality is fairly strictly defined as unchanging. If changeable dispositions such as coping strategies are considered, of course, the literature is very large.

It would have been enormously helpful, at the onset of the AIDS epidemic, to have had available the results of decades of well-supported sex research, just as it was of inestimable value to have previously funded an extremely competent biomedical research establishment. When AIDS burst upon the scene, we already had retrovirologists "ready" to identify HIV as a retrovirus. But when it became clear that AIDS was often passed on by sexual behaviors, we had no sexologists specializing in understanding anal sex, or "dry sex" among IV drug users, or the sexual habits of people with hemophilia. Although a few pioneers had begun to investigate such questions in the gay community (Carrier, 1976, 1977; Ross, 1986), their work was not accorded sufficient notice early in the epidemic when it would have been of great benefit. Accordingly, we have been crippled in the fight against AIDS on the behavioral front, and doubtless many have died as a result of our society's reluctance to fund studies to dispel our ignorance of sexual matters.

Similarly, there has been very little effort to "segment the market" for anal sex. Suppose that one group of gay men, ordinarily indifferent to anal sex, perform it because their partners very much prefer it–but also enjoy a wide variety of other sexual acts. And suppose that another group strongly prefers receptive anal sex over all other methods of achieving orgasm ("anything else is just foreplay"). Even though it would be best for both groups to eliminate unprotected anal sex, a factually-based, frequency-reduction campaign would probably succeed better with the first group, and an eroticization-of-condoms campaign would probably fare better with the latter. Even though we acknowledge that safer sex campaigns must be targeted to different groups in different ways (injecting drug users, black homosexual men, women, people with hemophilia, young heterosexuals, etc.), we do not seem to know how to target different subtypes of all the above (women who believe that they must obey their husbands, gay men with strong submissive fantasies, people with hemophilia who are emotionally exhausted from a lifetime of medical procedures, etc.).

Our research group is attempting to identify and characterize erotic subtypes of gay men in a series of papers, of which this is one. In a previous paper, we showed (see below) that depression is more common in gay men with gender nonconforming childhoods than in other gay men. Because such a childhood has been associated with a higher rate of receptive anal sex (at least before the AIDS epidemic–Weinrich, Grant, Jacobson, Robinson, McCutchan, & the HNRC Group, 1992), we may wish to target certain interventions directly at this subgroup. In another study (see below), we showed how certain MMPI personality variables correlated with unsafe sex and with an escape-avoidant coping style; this style was in turn associated with higher lifetime rates of bisexuality. Although we could of course make no inferences about the direction of causality, this second study underscored the likelihood that there are deeper reasons why some men prefer certain sexual acts–reasons which are highly relevant to the design of safer-sex campaigns in the face of this epidemic.

PREVIOUS RESULTS

We are fortunate to be associated with a research project concerning a large ($n > 500$) population of men, the majority homosexual or bisexual, from whom we have already gathered data on sexual behavior, coping styles, personality, depression, and femininity. The HIV Neurobehavioral Research Center is a large, federally-funded interdisciplinary research project affiliated with the Department of Psychiatry at the University of California, San Diego, and two local hospitals. Its basic mission is to investigate the natural history and prevalence of the neuropsychological sequelae of HIV infection, with attention being given to psychiatry, psychology, sexology, neurology, virology, medicine, brain imaging, and other disciplines. In two previous papers, we reported data from a variety of variables gathered from the gay/bisexual portion of our sample. In this paper, we see if these results are confirmed in an enlarged sample, and how they break down by HIV serostatus.

In Study 1 (Weinrich, Atkinson, Grant, & the HNRC Group, 1992; Weinrich, Atkinson, Grant, & the HNRC Group, 1994, in press), we demonstrated that:

> (1) Adult gay men who reported highly gender-nonconforming childhoods were more likely than those reporting more conforming childhoods to have current symptoms of anxiety and depression by self-report, and to have had a lifetime history of depression by clinical interview–depression which in nearly all cases preceded the

AIDS epidemic. The subscale measuring core gender identity nonconformity (or so-called "gender dysphoria") was more often associated with depression and anxiety than were the factors measuring other types of childhood gender nonconformity.

In Study 2 (Weinrich, Atkinson, Patterson, McCutchan, Gonsiorek, Grant et al., 1993; Weinrich, Patterson, Atkinson, McCutchan, Gonsiorek, Grant et al., 1994, in preparation), we used canonical correlation analyses of MMPI-2, Klein Grid, sex history, and Coping questionnaires to show that:

(2) A coping style characterized by high Escape-Avoidant and low Confrontive coping is associated with a higher likelihood to have identified one's past or ideal sexual orientation as more heterosexual than it was at time of interview. That is, bisexual or homosexual men who would prefer to be heterosexual, or who were more heterosexual in the past, are also more likely to show an Escape-Avoidant coping profile in nonsexual contexts.

(3) There are personality types which are associated with different patterns of safer-sex rejection:

(3a) A man who is socially inept, aloof, withdrawn, or anxious, who often acts out yet blames others for his problems (externalizes), or who gets into trouble due to a lack of internal controls yet gets caught because he is insufficiently devious, was more likely than the other gay men in our sample to move toward *un*safe sex in the period from 1984 to 1989. (Or less likely to move in the direction of safer sex.) Some of these men were celibate (perhaps not yet out of the closet) in 1984; for these men, this pattern reflects one in which they began their gay sex lives with more unsafe sex than was typical in our sample.

(3b) A man who is deeply conflicted, self-punishing, self-destructive, painfully disturbed, and troubled in coping with everything in life was more likely than other gay men in our sample to show a consistent pattern of unsafe sex in both 1984 and 1989.

In order to understand the results of Study 2 and our refinement of them in the present paper, some background information about canonical correlation is useful. (Readers familiar with canonical correlation who understand its application in the results reported above can skip to the last paragraph of this section.) In this type of analysis, one set of related variables (call them X variables) is correlated against a second set of variables (Y variables). The statistical procedure constructs two linear combinations, called canonical variables (CVs), one for the Xs and one for the Ys. These linear combinations can be thought of as recipes (this much of X_1, that much of X_2), but the weights can be positive or negative. Accordingly, CVs can turn out to be contrast variables, weighted sums, or a combination–indeed, any possible linear combination of the underlying set of variables.

The CV for the X variables and the CV for the Y variables are mathematically constructed to maximize the correlation between the two. Once this pair of CVs is ascertained, the canonical correlation procedure removes the variance associated with them from the dataset and then searches for a second pair of linear combinations of the X and Y variables with maximum correlation. By design, they are mathematically independent of the first pair. It continues this process until the degrees of freedom are exhausted, and provides statistical tests to tell investigators whether the CVs identified may be interpreted. Canonical correlation is especially useful when investigators suspect that there may be relationships between groups of variables which would not be revealed by a series of simple correlations.

In Study 2, we performed two canonical correlations. In the first, the X variables were the 13 t-scores from the MMPI-2 (see Methods), and the Y variables were our measure of unsafe sex (RSR: receiving semen rectally without a condom) at two time periods (pre- and post-AIDS). We found that there were two significant pairs of CVs for the first analysis, listed in 3a and 3b above. The second canonical correlation's X variables were the 8 Ways of Coping factor scores, and the Y variables were the 5 Klein Grid scores. Here we found one significant CV pair. This is result 2 above.

In the present paper, we seek to discover whether HIV serostatus affects the results we have previously reported. For study 1, that means that we will not primarily seek new correlations between childhood femininity and adult depression, but will see if the earlier findings are replicated in each HIV-status subgroup. For study 2, we do not report new canonical variables, but rather investigate whether the correlations previously observed in the sample as a whole continue to hold true for the HIV positive and HIV negative subsamples separately. In the following Methods subsection we will be brief because these details have been previously reported.

METHODS

Subjects: Both Studies

The universe from which each sample was drawn consisted of over 500 gay or bisexual men in the San Diego HIV Neurobehavioral Research

Center (HNRC). In this sample are HIV positive and negative men recruited from two sources: homosexual and bisexual men from San Diego's gay community, and the HIV program of a large local hospital (recruited without regard to sexual orientation; only the homosexual and bisexual men are considered in the present report). Inclusion/exclusion criteria for the subjects in the parent study were: aged 18-49 at entry to study, having more than 9 years of education, without a diagnosis of AIDS Dementia Complex at entry, not an injecting drug user, and without medical problems which might complicate the interpretation of a neuropsychological profile (e.g., Huntington's Disease, diabetes, or head injury). Typical participants had some college education, were in their thirties at time of entry into the study, and were Caucasian non-Hispanics. Hispanics and African-Americans each constituted about 8% of the sample.

Procedures: Both Studies

All questionnaires were mailed to a subject about a week before his baseline visit, with the exception of the MMPI-2 (which was added to the battery relatively recently and was sometimes obtained at a subsequent visit). During the Medical Core portion of the visit, the subject's answers to the sex history questionnaire and Klein Sexual Orientation Grid were examined for completeness and consistency. Any problems or ambiguities were cleared up in a face-to-face interview before the end of the visit. The MMPI-2 was retrieved by the Psychiatry Core during its visit with the subject, and the Ways of Coping questionnaire was collected by the HNRC's Life Events Project. The FGI questionnaire was scored using the HyperCard program, then transferred to the main databanks. MMPI-2 answer sheets were sent to a commercial service for scoring; the resultant t-scores were then entered into the database. Data were eventually transferred to the JMP statistical program from the SAS Institute.

Methods, Procedures, and Previous Analyses: Study 1

To qualify for Study 1, subjects must have completed the FGI questionnaire and have usable scores for at least one of the depression variables under study. Also excluded were two individuals with extremely high FGI scores (see Weinrich et al., 1992, for the exclusion rationale). Because the sample sizes involved in the breakdowns would have in some cases dropped below 50, we added newly qualifying cases to the data presented here. (There were no significant changes in the findings.) The result was a sample size ranging from 370 to 418, depending upon the *ns* of other variables available for each analysis.

We administered the Freund Feminine Gender Identity scale (FGI; Freund, Langevin, Satterberg, & Steiner, 1977) and a self-report measure of psychiatric symptoms (Profile of Mood States, or POMS–McNair, Lorr, & Droppleman, 1980). We chose to analyze two scores from the POMS for that report: Depression/Dejection and Tension/Anxiety. Subjects also underwent a standard, face-to-face diagnostic psychiatric interview (the Structured Clinical Interview for DSM-III-R, or SCID–Spitzer, Williams, Gibbon, & First, 1988), from which we analyzed the diagnoses of SCID Major Depression, Lifetime, and Major Depression, Current.

New Analyses: Study 1

Some gay men undergo a period of depression in their teenage years or in later life as they face the fact that their sexual orientation is disapproved by much of society. Such depression would have been included in the Lifetime diagnosis. We added the SCID variable of Major Depression, Current to the analyses as a measure of how much the depression persisted into the adult period, even though this was not reported in the original study.

We used Wilcoxon/Kruskal-Wallis tests (so-called non-parametric ANO-VAs) and contingency tables (Fisher's exact test) to analyze whether our HIV positive and negative subsamples differed on any of our depression variables. Then we performed logistic regressions for each of these variables against total FGI score–separately for the two HIV serostatus groups. Resultant Ns were 417-418 for the POMS analyses and 370 for the SCID.

Methods, Procedures, and Previous Analyses: Study 2

To qualify for Study 2, subjects had to have had sex with another man at least once by 1989, and to have completed enough procedures at the baseline visit to provide us with data on at least two of the four major variables under study. Between 271 and 378 men qualified, depending upon the analysis.

We administered the Ways of Coping Scale–Revised (Folkman & Lazarus, 1988), the revised edition of the Minnesota Multiphasic Personality Inventory (MMPI-2; Hathaway, McKinley, Butcher, Dahlstrom, Graham, & Tellegen, 1989), the Klein Sexual Orientation Grid (KSOG; Klein, Sepekoff, & Wolf, 1985), and a sex history questionnaire devised by the HNRC Medical Core (for reliability and validity of this instrument, see Weinrich, Jacobson, Robinson, Grant, the HNRC Group, & McCutchan, 1994).

The MMPI-2 scoring produced the usual 10 clinical and 3 interpretative scale scores. The Ways of Coping Scale also has a standard scoring, which produces 8 factor scores representing different coping styles (Escape-avoidant, Confrontive, Seek Social Support, Distancing, Self-Controlling, Accept Responsibility, Problem Solving, and Positive Reappraisal). As our index of safer sex we chose a behavior which is highly unsafe if one does not know the serostatus of one's sexual partner: receiving semen rectally without a condom (RSR). This behavior was assessed by the sex history questionnaire at several time periods, of which we chose two: the pre-safer-sex period of 1979-1984, and 1989 (the most recent period in which we had complete information for all of our subjects). Frequency was assessed on a six-point scale (where 1 = "Never" in this time period and 6 = "Usually" in this time period). Subjects were provided with percentage ranges defining each of the 6 intervals while completing the questionnaire.

An early factor analysis of the Klein Grid on the HNRC sample (Weinrich, Snyder, Pillard, Grant, Jacobson, Robinson et al., 1993) was revised (Weinrich et al., 1994, in preparation) because the number of subjects available for the present study was much larger. The factors from the more recent analysis are used here, and summarized in Figure 1. As is common in factor analysis, when the sample was enlarged some of the previously identified factors split into smaller, more focused factors. For example, the general sexual orientation factor identified in the smaller study became three factors in the larger study, which we have named Past Sexual Orientation, Present Sexual Orientation, and Ideal Sexual Orientation. Each of these is heavily loaded upon by 4 of the 21 Klein items. The smaller study's "contrast" factor (in which all 14 Present and Past sexual orientation items loaded positively, and all 7 Ideal items loaded negatively) disappeared because Past, Present, and Ideal sexual orientations are now separate factors in the larger analysis. (Tellingly–and reassuringly–this contrast re-emerged in the canonical correlations.) The Social factor of the smaller analysis was joined by the Emotional items in the larger one.

Results from the previous analyses of these canonical correlations were reported in a previous section. In addition, we showed in Study 2 that the Escape-Avoidant Coping CV was modestly correlated in the expected direction with each of the two CVs of the MMPI-2, thus establishing an indirect link among all four CVs.

New Analyses: Study 2

For the present paper, we split the sample into HIV positive and negative subgroups, and first examined whether their scores differed on the

FIGURE 1. Klein Sexual Orientation Grid (KSOG) Factor Structure

SA: Sexually attracted to:	Past	Pres	Ideal	
SB: Sexual behavior; has/had sex with:	Past	Pres	Ideal	0 = other sex only
SF: Sexual fantasies involve:	Past	Pres	Ideal	3 = both equally
Em: Emotionally close to:	EmSoc	EmSoc	EmSoc	6 = own sex only
SP: Social preference/socialize with:	EmSoc	EmSoc	EmSoc	
ID: Self identification as:	Past	Pres	Ideal	0 = heterosexual/s only
LS: Lifestyle/spend time with:	LS	LS	LS	3 = both equally
	Past	Now	Ideally	6 = homosexual/s only

Key:

Past: Past Sexual Orientation factor

Pres: Present Sexual Orientation factor

Ideal: Ideal Sexual Orientation factor

EmSoc: Emotional/Social factor

LS: Lifestyle factor

three pairs of canonical variables (primarily by ANOVA and t-test, but checked by the nonparametric Wilcoxon/Kruskal-Wallis test). Then we used simple linear regressions to see if the relationship detected for the sample as a whole was replicated in each subgroup.

RESULTS

Study 1

Comparisons between our HIV positive and negative subjects on the depression variables are shown in Table 1. Strictly speaking, there are no significant differences between the groups, but HIV positives scored perhaps a little higher on POMS Tension/Anxiety ($p = 0.06$) and Major Depression, Recent ($p < 0.07$ in a one-tailed Fisher's exact test, but only a weak trend, $p < 0.13$, in a two-tailed test).

Results of the analyses assessing the relationship between FGI score and the POMS scores (by HIV status) are presented in Figures 2 and 3, which show that the associations are modestly strengthened or un-

TABLE 1. Depression by HIV Serostatus

Wilcoxon/Kruskal-Wallis Tests

	n	Mean Rank	Chi-Square approximation χ^2	DF	p
POMS Depression/Dejection					
HIV+	399	248	0.002	1	0.97
HIV−	96	249			
POMS Tension/Anxiety					
HIV+	398	253	3.53	1	0.06
HIV−	96	223			

Fisher's Exact Tests

	No	Yes	Fisher's Exact Tests 1-tail p	2-tail p
Major Depression at Interview				
HIV+	345	38	0.07	0.13
HIV−	74	3		
Major Depression Lifetime				
HIV+	237	146	0.20	0.38
HIV−	43	34		

Note: Sixteen individuals who were initially recruited to the HNRC via a treatment program for clinically depressed HIV positive men were excluded from this table. Obviously, to include them would have biased the breakdowns reported here. These subjects' data were not eliminated from the other tables, which report analyses attempting to discern the relationship between depression and other variables.

changed in the HIV positive subsample, but are nonexistent in the HIV negative subsample. When significant, p values are highly so (p < 0.005), although the proportions of the variance explained by the FGI score are modest. Exploratory analyses are underway to see if this relationship is mostly due, as the original finding was, to the Core Gender Identity factor of the FGI.

Precisely the same conclusions can be drawn from the logistic regression analyses showing the relationship between the FGI score and the lifetime SCID depression score (by HIV status) presented in Figure 4. The association–in which high-FGI men are more likely to be diagnosed with

FIGURE 2. POMS Depression/Dejection as a Function of FGI Score

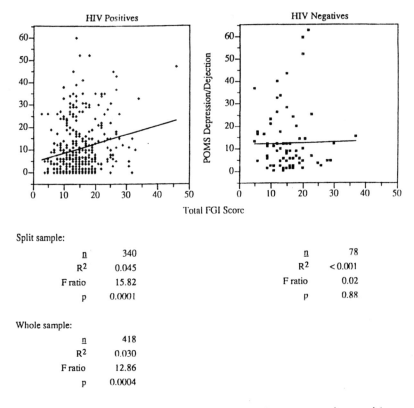

Split sample:

n	340	n	78
R^2	0.045	R^2	< 0.001
F ratio	15.82	F ratio	0.02
p	0.0001	p	0.88

Whole sample:

n	418
R^2	0.030
F ratio	12.86
p	0.0004

SCID Major Depression, Lifetime, disappears for seronegatives, with unambiguous p-values on both sides.

Because only 4 HIV negative subjects were diagnosed as depressed at time of initial interview, we can only present data on FGI score and current depression for the HIV positive sample and the sample as a whole (Figure 5). Again, the finding persists unambiguously in the HIV positive subsample.

Study 2

First, we examined whether HIV status was correlated with scores on any of the three pairs of CVs originally identified in Study 2. Results are shown in Table 2. Four of the six CVs were not significantly associated with HIV status (all *ps* > 0.15). For one variable, the Escape-Avoidant Coping CV, the HIV positive group showed a trend toward a higher

FIGURE 3. POMS Tension/Anxiety as a Function of FGI Score

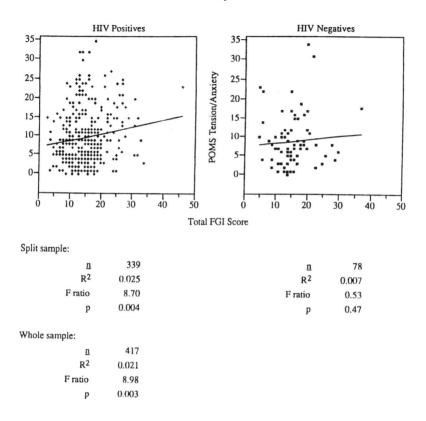

Split sample:

	n	339
	R^2	0.025
	F ratio	8.70
	p	0.004

	n	78
	R^2	0.007
	F ratio	0.53
	p	0.47

Whole sample:

	n	417
	R^2	0.021
	F ratio	8.98
	p	0.003

amount of this kind of coping ($p < 0.07$). There was a significant ($p < 0.01$) tendency for the HIV positive group to score higher on a pattern in which unsafe sex is high both before and after the epidemic. Results are essentially unchanged if nonparametric tests are used (data not presented here).

Results of our breakdowns of CV correlations by HIV status are presented in Figures 6 to 8. In two of the three cases, the pattern is clear and replicates the results presented earlier in this paper: the correlations we observed in the sample as a whole are confirmed in each of the HIV positive subsamples, but do not reach significance in the HIV negative subsamples. The finding for the second pair of CVs on the MMPI/Safer Sex side (Figure 7) are significant for the sample as a whole, but drop to only trend levels of significance ($p < 0.15$ and $p < 0.09$) when broken down by HIV status.

FIGURE 4. SCID Major Depression Lifetime as a Function of FGI Score

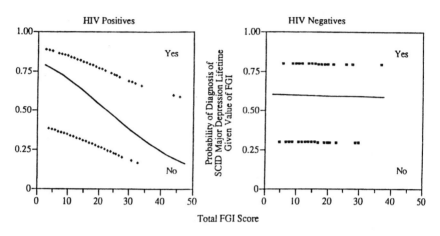

Guide to interpretation of the charts above:

In a logistic regression, a dichotomous dependent variable (diagnosis of depression) is predicted by a continuous independent variable (FGI). The curve represents the probability, as it varies by FGI score, of the dependent variable being true (depressed). In the left-hand chart, the curve slopes sharply downward, indicating that a diagnosis of depression is much more likely for those with high FGI scores than without. The horizontal position of each point represents a particular individual with that FGI score. Its vertical position has no significance, except to indicate whether that person has the diagnosis (above the curve) or does not (below).

Split sample:

	n	312		n	57
	R^2	0.030		R^2	< 0.0001
	χ^2	12.36		χ^2	< 0.01
	p	0.0005		p	0.97

Whole sample:

	n	370
	R^2	0.021
	χ^2	10.38
	p	0.002

Even though the HIV negative group typically did not replicate the canonical correlations of the first study, the correlations of the Escape-Avoidant CV with the two MMPI CVs were replicated in *both* subsamples (Figures 9-10). Moreover, in both cases the strength of the association between the regressed variables (as measured by R^2) was over twice

FIGURE 5. SCID Current Depression as a Function of FGI Score

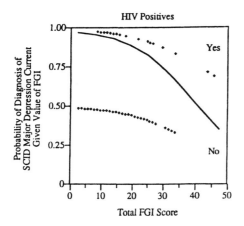

For interpretation of the logistic regression chart above, see Figure 4.

HIV positive sample:

n	313	
R^2	0.065	
χ^2	12.52	
p	0.0005	

Because there are only 4 HIV negative subjects with this diagnosis, no correlation will be provided.

Whole sample:

n	370
R^2	0.062
χ^2	13.17
p	0.0003

as strong for the HIV negatives than for the HIV positives! This is a remarkable reversal, given the large discrepancy in the sizes of the two groups.

DISCUSSION

Depression and Childhood Gender Nonconformity

In our earlier paper on depression and gender nonconformity (Weinrich et al., 1992; Weinrich et al., 1994, in press), some readers may have

TABLE 2. Canonical Variable (CV) Scores by HIV Status

Variable	Total n	*n* or Mean HIV+	*n* or Mean HIV–	t-test	p
<u>Sexual Behavior CVs</u>	491	395	96		
Moved toward safer sex		0.063	0.069	0.60	0.55
Consistently unsafe sex		0.147	0.124	2.74	0.01
<u>MMPI CVs</u>	336	257	79		
Externalizing/Incompetent Sociopath		0.238	0.252	1.44	0.16
General MMPI Psychopathology		0.672	0.663	0.92	0.36
<u>Klein Grid CV</u>	478	383	95		
Ideal/Past/Present					
Sexual Orientation Consistency		–0.0019	0.0042	1.002	0.32
<u>Coping CV</u>	400	309	91		
Escape-avoidant coping style		0.037	0.026	1.823	0.07

interpreted our results as a general statement about all subgroups of gay men: that those who had gender nonconforming childhoods, especially if they were gender dysphoric, were in general more likely to have depressive episodes persisting well into, or throughout, adulthood. However, we have just reported that this finding holds only in our HIV positive subsample, not our negative controls.

Care must be taken in interpreting this finding. Since the depression nearly always first manifested itself before the HIV era, it is difficult to argue that HIV seropositive men who are highly gender nonconforming are more likely to be depressed (because of their HIV status) than HIV negative men who are highly gender nonconforming. But there is no significant difference in the incidence of lifetime depression by HIV status anyway (Table 1), nor in depressive symptomatology at baseline (as measured by the POMS subscale).

One might suggest that the gay men who were the most gender dysphoric were the ones most likely to jump quickly and uncritically into receptive anal sex (seeing that act consciously or unconsciously as a quintessentially feminine act), a hypothesis which has some modest empirical support (Weinrich et al., 1992). They thus would have been more likely to be exposed to HIV early in their sexual careers, and would have been

FIGURE 6. HIV Status Effects on Correlation Between Personality and Unsafe Sex (Part 1)

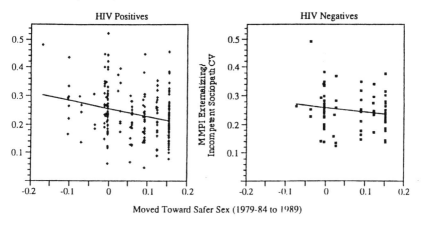

Split sample:

n	231		n	75
R^2	0.078		R^2	0.028
F ratio	19.48		F ratio	2.11
p	< 0.0001		p	0.15

Whole sample:

n	306
R^2	0.067
F ratio	21.87
p	< 0.0001

disproportionately depleted from the HIV negative control group. There is some evidence for this in Figures 2 and 3, where examination of the scatterplots reveals much wider scatter on the seropositive sides. But in Figure 4, only a handful of HIV positives were far beyond the main mass of HIV negative scores.

Personality and Safer Sex

In our other previous investigation (Weinrich et al., 1993; Weinrich et al., 1994, in preparation), we were searching for some of the deeper reasons why some gay men continue to engage in unsafe sex in the face of a lethal epidemic. Of course, the dangers of unprotected receptive anal intercourse

FIGURE 7. HIV Status Effects on Correlation Between Personality and Unsafe Sex (Part 2)

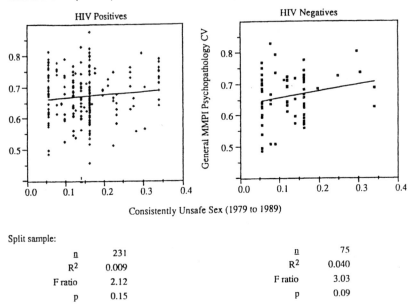

Split sample:

$\underline{n}$	231
R^2	0.009
F ratio	2.12
p	0.15

$\underline{n}$	75
R^2	0.040
F ratio	3.03
p	0.09

Whole sample:

$\underline{n}$	306
R^2	0.015
F ratio	4.78
p	0.03

are different for HIV negatives and positives. The former risk getting the disease itself; the latter risk (at most) reinfection from a more virulent strain.

Viewed from this perspective, the two variables identified from the MMPI-2 scores are especially interesting. The first represents a tendency to move to more unsafe sex from the time period before AIDS to after AIDS, or at least a tendency to "come out" with a pattern of unsafe sex as one begins one's sexual career in the gay community (at a time when one is presumably HIV negative). This dangerous pattern, according to our previous study, is associated with a personality profile suggesting that one resists society's "do-gooder" messages or has a tendency to get oneself unnecessarily into trouble. This pattern clearly persisted for the HIV positives, but weakened or disappeared for the HIV negatives. Examination of the scatterplots in

FIGURE 8. HIV Status Effects on Correlation Between Coping Style and Sexual Orientation Ambivalence

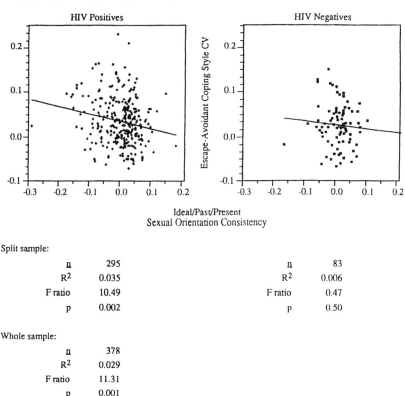

Split sample:					
	n	295		n	83
	R^2	0.035		R^2	0.006
	F ratio	10.49		F ratio	0.47
	p	0.002		p	0.50

Whole sample:		
	n	378
	R^2	0.029
	F ratio	11.31
	p	0.001

Figure 6 show that the greater variability in both dependent and independent variables on the HIV positive side is probably not merely due to the larger *n*. First–and not surprisingly–the HIV negative scatterplot essentially lacks a left-hand (unsafe sex) side. Second, both subsamples show a concentration in the lower right quadrant, but the HIV positive scatterplot is also heavy in the upper left. This quadrant may contain a group of gay men whose personalities are especially prone to ignore safer-sex messages.

One interpretation is that any HIV negatives who show such a pattern will quickly move into the HIV positive group. For example, gay men newly coming out, and having unsafe sex, will be more likely to encounter our study after seroconversion than before. Another sample selection bias could be influencing these results if we hypothesize that men who are

FIGURE 9. MMPI CVs as a Function of Escape-Avoidant Coping CV (Part 1)

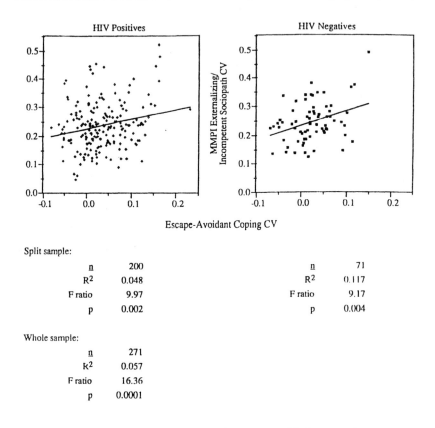

Split sample:

n	200		n	71
R²	0.048		R²	0.117
F ratio	9.97		F ratio	9.17
p	0.002		p	0.004

Whole sample:

n	271
R²	0.057
F ratio	16.36
p	0.0001

suspicious of society's health campaigns are unlikely to volunteer as a control for a study as complicated as ours.

A very similar pattern is seen in the analyses of the Klein Grid canonical variable and the Escape-Avoidant CV (Figure 8). The significant correlation between the two remains (or is strengthened) when confined to the HIV positive subsample, and disappears in the HIV negative controls. As in the previous instance, examination of the scatterplots shows that both groups cluster near the origin or "average" (0, 0), but the HIV positive group disperses far more into the quadrant which strengthens the association. Again, there are at least two plausible interpretations: that the men who are high on Escape-Avoidance will move quickly into the HIV positive group (which seems less likely to occur *a priori* in this instance), or that such men are less likely to volunteer for a complicated

FIGURE 10. MMPI CVs as a Function of Escape-Avoidant Coping CV (Part 2)

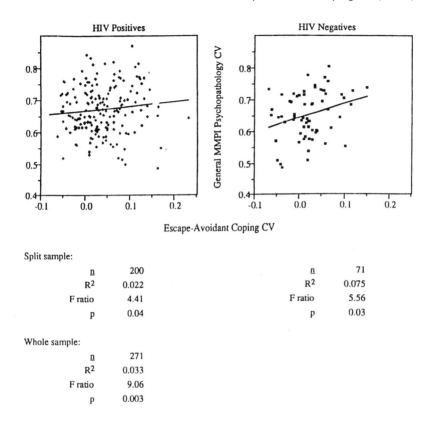

Split sample:

n	200		n	71
R^2	0.022		R^2	0.075
F ratio	4.41		F ratio	5.56
p	0.04		p	0.03

Whole sample:

n	271
R^2	0.033
F ratio	9.06
p	0.003

study such as ours if their Escape-Avoidance has somehow managed to keep them HIV negative. If Escape-Avoidance has "worked" for you, why join a study in which you have to confront the possibility that you might seroconvert?

Figures 9 and 10 are interesting because they show a consistent pattern with each other but a different pattern from the earlier findings: the associations detected in the sample as a whole remain significant in both HIV positive and HIV negative subgroups. This suggests that this association reflects an underlying psychological principle: namely, that people who tend to employ an escape-avoidant coping style are more likely to blame others for their difficulties, to do so in a way which is sometimes self-injurious, and may reflect deeper psychological problems. This suggests continuing vigilance as we can follow these men prospectively to see if they are more likely to move toward more unsafe behaviors–or even to seroconvert (but see the next section).

The second MMPI pattern, with a "recipe" which correlates significantly with 9 of the 10 clinical MMPI scales, correlated in our original study with a consistent tendency to perform unsafe sex both pre- and post-AIDS. This correlation persisted significantly in the enlarged total sample, but weakened into insignificance in both serostatus groups (Figure 7). As before, there is much more variation in the unsafe sex variable for the HIV positives than for the controls. But there is not much difference in the scatter on the MMPI side. As we receive prospective reports of the behavior of the six controls who scored high on this MMPI variable, we may derive further insights into the typical histories followed by such men.

Follow-Up of Highly At-Risk Individuals

In a study such as ours, we have the opportunity to observe patterns which may have been involved in HIV exposure for our seropositive subjects. Some of these patterns have been reported in the present paper. But there are exceptions to the general rule: men who share those patterns but who remain seronegative, because they have not had enough time to undergo the experiences which may cause them to be exposed in the future, because they are at less risk than they seem to be at because of other factors not considered in our models, or because they just have enjoyed good luck.

Our study is also longitudinal, so we have the intellectual option to sit back and watch to see if our hypotheses, derived from cross-sectional analyses, will prove true over time as some fraction of the highest-risk individuals make their mistakes and seroconvert. Again keeping a large, clinical distance, we may speculate that our correlations will become statistically less troublesome in a few years.

We are, to put it mildly and a bit sarcastically, reluctant to discuss how stimulating such carefully controlled follow-up could be. In the past year (as of this writing), the senior author of this paper has seen two personal acquaintances with just such a personality pattern seroconvert–individuals he had hoped and expected would remain permanent, seronegative exceptions to the rules he was discovering in this research. No one who has had such an experience can, in good conscience, just sit back and let nature take its course. In concordance with most AIDS prevention workers, we would like to identify such men and find a way to reach them before seroconversion.

Lives *will* be saved if we can succeed in such efforts, even if the task continues to be difficult. All of us involved in AIDS research need to face the fact that there are at-risk individuals in the real world who will resist safer-sex messages of the ordinary, these-are-the-facts type, just as we know that not everyone cares about *Consumer Reports*. More subtle campaigns will be needed, perhaps ones which strike emotional rather than rational chords in the target audience. Condom use as an act of rebellion might be a good theme to start with.

Broader Implications

Our results have important implications for behavioral scientists and those involved in AIDS research and prevention. First, we repeat our warning that denial kills–or at least (as represented by Escape-Avoidant coping) is correlated with personality types which have high levels of unsafe sex (Figures 9 and 10). The fact that this finding persists for both MMPI variables even in the HIV negative subsamples underscores this danger.

Our results also suggest that other personality and dispositional variables play a role in the steps leading to the adoption of safer sex practices, but that this role is measurable mostly in the HIV positive group. The consistency of this finding in several different domains is remarkable, and we are somewhat dissatisfied with the lack of parsimony in our efforts to explain these results. In each case, it seemed, we were invoking a different kind of plausible but unproven sample selection bias.

But what if this consistency is trying to tell us something? Perhaps this finding is much more than a collection of sampling peculiarities. Given that many HIV negative men have led sex lives indistinguishable from their gay friends who are now seropositive, and now that the biomedical researchers are showing that there are immune system responses (especially in the cellular half of the immune system) which apparently offer some protection against HIV exposure, there is a very real possibility that a substantial proportion of the HIV negatives are genetically predisposed, through the operation of their personality or their immune chemistry, to avoid or resist infection by HIV. If this daring hypothesis is correct, it could explain all of our findings pertaining to correlations with the MMPI-2 unsafe-sex variables. We recommend that further studies should immediately be undertaken to see if there are any immune system correlates of personality variables or other personal characteristics which might affect one's likelihood of acquiring an HIV infection. This clearly speculative hypothesis, if confirmed, would have highly significant consequences for the entire field of biopsychosocial aspects of AIDS.

In the mid-1980s, when gay men were first identified as a major risk group for AIDS (and before the involvement of other risk groups was apparent), the senior author was often asked if gay men might be more likely to come down with AIDS for some genetic reason, perhaps a genetic reason involved in their becoming gay in the first place. He always replied that although this was a theoretical possibility, it was on its face an extremely remote one. After all, what kind of gene could be imagined which would not only affect sexual orientation, particular sexual preferences, and immune system parameters all at once?

With the recent identification of a genetic marker for homosexuality on the X chromosome (Hamer, Hu, Magnuson, Hu, & Pattatucci, 1993), pioneering reports of immune system correlates of particular genitoerotic preferences in gay men (Ross, 1986), and a theory which might predict a causal connection between sexual orientation and immune functioning (Geschwind & Galaburda, 1985 a, b, c), this picture may be changing in the near future. If so, it could imply that we might not even expect to see similarities between HIV positive and HIV negative gay men in analyses such as those as we have investigated here. Of course, heterosexuals are perfectly capable of contracting AIDS through sexual contact, so we should not expect any simplistic homosexual/heterosexual dichotomies to prevail (as might have been in the minds of the questioners mentioned above). But if there are subtypes of homosexuals and heterosexuals who are more or less likely to contract HIV for any reasons other than the obviously behavioral ones, dismissing such possibilities out of hand may turn out to be anything from intellectually unfortunate to medically fatal.

NOTE

1. The HNRC Group includes: Igor Grant, MD, Director; J. Hampton Atkinson, MD, Co-Director; Robert A. Velin, PhD, Center Manager; Edward C. Oldfield III, MD, James L. Chandler, MD, Mark R. Wallace, MD, and Joseph Malone, MD, Co-Investigators Naval Hospital San Diego; J. Allen McCutchan, MD, PI Medical Core; Stephen A. Spector, MD, PI Virology Core; Leon Thal, MD, PI Neurology Core; Robert K. Heaton, PhD, PI Neuropsychology Core; John Hesselink, MD and Terry Jernigan, PhD, Co-PIs Imaging Core; J. Hampton Atkinson, MD, PI Psychiatry Core; Clayton A. Wiley, MD, PhD, PI Neuropathology Core; Richard Olshen, PhD and Ian Abramson, PhD, Co-PIs Biostatistics Core; Nelson Butters, PhD, PI Memory Project; Renée Dupont, MD, PI SPECT Project; Thomas Patterson, PhD, PI Life Events Project; Sidney Zisook, MD, PI Mood Project; Dilip Jeste, MD, PI Psychosis Project; Hans Sieburg, PhD, PI Dynamical Systems Project; and James D. Weinrich, PhD, PI Sexology Project.

REFERENCES

Carrier, J. M. (1976). Cultural factors affecting urban Mexican male homosexual behavior. *Archives of Sexual Behavior, 5,* 103-124.

Carrier, J. M. (1977). "Sex-role preference" as an explanatory variable in homosexual behavior. *Archives of Sexual Behavior, 6,* 53-65.

Clement, U. (1992). Psychological correlates of unprotected intercourse among HIV-positive gay men. *Journal of Psychology & Human Sexuality, 5*(1-2), 133- 155.

Folkman, S., & Lazarus, R. (1988). *Ways of Coping Revised Questionnaire.* Palo Alto CA: Consulting Psychologists Press.

Freund, K. W., Langevin, R., Satterberg, J., & Steiner, B. W. (1977). Extension of the feminine gender identity for males. *Archives of Sexual Behavior, 6,* 507-519.

Geschwind, N., & Galaburda, A. M. (1985a). Cerebral lateralization: Biological mechanisms, associations, and pathology: I. A hypothesis and a program for research. *Archives of Neurology, 42,* 428-459.

Geschwind, N., & Galaburda, A. M. (1985b). Cerebral lateralization: Biological mechanisms, associations, and pathology: II. A hypothesis and a program for research. *Archives of Neurology, 42,* 521-552.

Geschwind, N., & Galaburda, A. M. (1985c). Cerebral lateralization: Biological mechanisms, associations, and pathology: III. A hypothesis and a program for research. *Archives of Neurology, 42,* 634-654.

Hamer, D. H., Hu, S., Magnuson, V. L., Hu, N., & Pattatucci, A. M. L. (1993). A linkage between DNA markers on the X chromosome and male sexual orientation. *Science, 261,* 321-327.

Hathaway, S. R., McKinley, J. C., Butcher, J. N., Dahlstrom, W. G., Graham, J. R., & Tellegen, A. (1989). MMPI-2: Minnesota Multiphasic Personality Inventory–2. Minneapolis MN: University of Minnesota Press.

Kelly, J. A., St. Lawrence, J. S., & Brasfield, T. L. (1990). Predictors of vulnerability to AIDS risk behavior relapse. *Journal of Social Psychology, 130,* 163-166.

Klein, F., Sepekoff, B., & Wolf, T. J. (1985). Sexual orientation: A multi-variable dynamic process. *Journal of Homosexuality, 11*(1/2), 35-49.

McCown, W. (1991). Contributions of the EPN paradigm to HIV prevention: A preliminary study. *Personality and Individual Differences, 12,* 1301-1303.

McCown, W. (1993). Personality factors predicting failure to practice safer sex by HIV positive males. *Personality and Individual Differences, 14,* 613-615.

McNair, D. M., Lorr, M., & Droppleman, L. F. (1980). *Profile of Mood States (POMS) manual.* San Diego CA: Educational and Industrial Testing Services.

Mosher, D. L. (1980). A three dimensional theory of depth of involvement in human sexual response. *Journal of Sex Research, 16,* 1-42.

Pakesch, G., Pfersmann, D., Loimer, N., Grunberger, J., Linzmayer, L., & Mayerhofer, S. (1992). [Noopsychological changes and psychopathological characteristics of HIV-1 patients of various risk groups]. *Fortschritte der Neurologie Psychiatrie, 60,* 17-27.

Ross, M. W. (1986). *Psychovenereology: Personality and lifestyles factors in sexually transmitted diseases in homosexual men.* New York: Praeger.

Ross, M. W. (1988). Personality factors that differentiate homosexual men with positive and negative attitudes toward condom use. *New York State Journal of Medicine, 88,* 626-628.

Ross, M. W. (1990). Psychovenereology: Psychological aspects of AIDS and other sexually transmissible diseases. In D. G. Ostrow (Ed.), *Behavioral aspects of AIDS* (pp. 19-40). New York: Plenum Medical Book Company.

Spitzer, R. L., Williams, J. B. W., Gibbon, M., & First, M. B. (1988). *Structured Clinical Interview for DSM-III-R (Nonpatient version)*. New York: New York State Psychiatric Institute.

Weinrich, J. D., Atkinson, J. H., Grant, I., & the HNRC Group (1992). Is gender dysphoria dysphoric? Elevated depression and anxiety in gender dysphoric but not other gender-nonconforming homosexual and bisexual men in an HIV sample. Annual meeting of the International Academy of Sex Research, Prague, July 8.

Weinrich, J. D., Atkinson, J. H., Grant, I., & the HNRC Group (1994). Is gender dysphoria dysphoric? Elevated depression and anxiety in gender dysphoric in comparison with other types of homosexual and bisexual men in an HIV sample. *Archives of Sexual Behavior, 23*,

Weinrich, J. D., Atkinson, J. H., Patterson, T. L., McCutchan, J. A., Gonsiorek, J. C., Grant, I., & the HNRC Group (1993). Unsafe sexual behavior predicted by MMPI-II personality scores and coping strategies. Annual meeting of the IX International Conference on AIDS, Berlin, p. 952.

Weinrich, J. D., Grant, I., Jacobson, D. L., Robinson, S. R., McCutchan, J. A., & the HNRC Group (1992). Effects of recalled childhood gender nonconformity on adult genitoerotic role and AIDS exposure. *Archives of Sexual Behavior, 21*, 559-585.

Weinrich, J. D., Jacobson, D. L., Robinson, S. R., Grant, I., the HNRC Group, & McCutchan, J. A. (1994). Reliability and validity of sex history information in an HIV sample, 1984-1992. *Archives of Sexual Behavior*, accepted for publication, pending submitted revisions.

Weinrich, J. D., Patterson, T. L., Atkinson, J. H., McCutchan, J. A., Gonsiorek, J. C., Grant, I., & the HNRC Group (1994, in preparation). Unsafe sexual behavior and conflict over sexual orientation as a function of escape/avoidant coping and MMPI-2 scores in a sample of homosexual and bisexual men.

Weinrich, J. D., Snyder, P. J., Pillard, R. C., Grant, I., Jacobson, D. L., Robinson, S. R., & McCutchan, J. A. (1993). A factor analysis of the Klein Sexual Orientation Grid in two disparate samples. *Archives of Sexual Behavior, 22*, 157-168.

HIV as a Catalyst for Positive Gay Men's Desire for Clarification, Enhancement and Promotion of Intimacy in Significant Relationships

Leslie Cannold, M. Bioethics
Bill O'Loughlin
Geoff Woolcock, BA
Brian Hickman, PhD

SUMMARY. Semi-structured interviews with fifteen HIV positive Australian men were conducted. Interviews explored the impact of HIV/AIDS on the participants' significant relationships. It was found that HIV had a catalytic effect on six (40%) of the participants' desires for clarification, enhancement and promotion of intimacy in their relationships with others. Of the six, four (66.7%) saw the locus of control for bringing about desired change in the degree of intimacy in their lives to lie within themselves, with two (33%) describing an external locus of control for the satisfaction of intimacy desires. The integration of the findings into Ross, Tebble and Viliunas' (1989) staged model of psychological reactions to HIV infection in asymptomatic homosexual men is discussed. *[Single or multiple copies of this*

Leslie Cannold, Bill O'Loughlin, Geoff Woolcock, and Brian Hickman are affiliated with the National Centre for HIV Social Research (Melbourne Unit), Melbourne, Victoria, Australia.

The authors gratefully acknowledge the contributions of Susie McLean, BA, and Beverly Raphael, AMM, MBBS, MD, FRANZCP, FASSA, FRCPsych, to this paper.

[Haworth co-indexing entry note]: "HIV as a Catalyst for Positive Gay Men's Desire for Clarification, Enhancement and Promotion of Intimacy in Significant Relationships." Cannold, Leslie et al. Co-published simultaneously in *Journal of Psychology & Human Sexuality* (The Haworth Press, Inc.) Vol. 7, No. 1/2, 1995, pp. 161-179; and: *HIV/AIDS and Sexuality* (ed: Michael W. Ross) The Haworth Press, Inc., 1995, pp. 161-179; and: *HIV/AIDS and Sexuality* (ed: Michael W. Ross) Harrington Park Press, an imprint of The Haworth Press, Inc., 1995, pp. 161-179. *[Single or multiple copies of this article are available from The Haworth Document Delivery Service: 1-800-342-9678, 9:00 a.m. - 5:00 p.m. (EST).]*

*article are available from The Haworth Document Delivery Service:
1-800-342-9678, 9:00 a.m. - 5:00 p.m. (EST).]*

INTRODUCTION

The relationships between social support and mental and physical well-being is well-documented (Kübler-Ross, 1969; Blythe, 1983; D'Augelli, 1993; Gottlieb, 1983; Ross, 1990; O'Brien, Wortmen, Kessler & Joseph, 1993; Turner, Hays & Coates, 1993). This relationship has been demonstrated in HIV positive gay men (Wolcott, Namir, Fawzy, Gottelieb & Mitsuyasu, 1986; Zich & Temoshok, 1987), as has the relationship between social support and positive gay identity (Hammersmith & Weinberg, 1973, Weinberg & Williams, 1974; Dannecker, 1981; Acevedo, 1986; Gonsiorek & Rudolph, 1991). Positive gay identity, in turn, has been related to psychological adjustment in gay men, (Hammersmith & Weinberg, 1973; Jacobs & Tedford, 1980; Schmitt & Kurdek, 1987a) and lower emotional distress in HIV positive gay men (Namir, Wolcott, Fawzy & Alumbaugh, 1987).

Berger (1990) notes that in the past decade, researchers have shifted their focus away from the sexual aspect of gay male couples to issues of love, commitment and affiliation (Peplau & Cochran, 1981; Blumstein & Schwartz, 1983; McWhirter & Mattison, 1984, Schmitt & Kurdek, 1987a, 1987b). Peplau (1991) reviewed research on gay and lesbian relationships and concluded that homosexual couples are largely similar in characteristics to heterosexual couples, and that gay men and lesbians strongly desire enduring close relationships. The majority of research on homosexual "relationships," however, has focused on romantic partnerships between homosexuals and between the homosexual couple and other significant persons (Kurdek & Schmitt, 1987b; Mattison & McWhirter, 1990). Researchers have only recently begun, using both quantitative and qualitative methods, to investigate the role played by the entire spectrum of significant relationships in the lives of individual gay men, and to ask about the impact of HIV on these relationships.

Nicholson and Long (1990) found that a positive attitude towards homosexuality is related to a greater use of problem-solving and support-seeking coping in HIV positive gay men. Schaeffer and Coleman, (1992), using a qualitative methodology, found that HIV positive gay men reported a shift in their sense of meaning, purpose and value after diagnosis. They also found that relationships, broadly defined, "brought the greatest sense of meaning, purpose and value." Minichiello's (1992) case studies of HIV positive gay men highlights the importance of support from men's families of origin and gay families. Minichiello refers to the "coming out" literature which focuses on "self-definition and public disclosure as important elements of identity formation," noting that participants in his research felt that disclosure of their HIV status was essential to, the words of one participant, their learning to "cope, to live with it." However, he emphasises the importance of the response to disclosure being supportive, encouraging, empathetic and non-judgmental in order for participants to experience "relief" from telling others. Turner, Hays and Coates' (1993) analyses of cross-sectional and longitudinal data on a probability sample of gay men in San Francisco (N = 1034) suggests the particular importance of communicating with family members about AIDS issues and maintaining positive feelings about being gay to support satisfaction. The authors note that approximately 50% of their study's population are presently infected with HIV.

What this research suggests is the contribution of social support and positive gay identity to the psychological well-being of HIV positive gay men. Social relationships of importance in the lives of HIV positive gay men include those with partners, families of origins, gay families and health care workers. A diagnosis of HIV seems to prompt in gay men a shift in the meaning and importance of relationships, and an attempt at resolution of unresolved issues around their homosexuality. The work suggests that the nature of the response of important others to disclosure impacts on the satisfaction gay men experience from telling others. However, further exploration of this suggestion, and the specific aspects of their relationships with others that positive gay men value is needed. The change gay men experience in the nature of their relationships with important others, and the desires they have for changing these relationships after a positive diagnosis also needs further study.

Kübler-Ross (1969) discusses five stages through which patients progress when facing a terminal illness: Denial and Isolation, Anger, Bargaining, Depression and Acceptance. Kübler-Ross (1987) notes that stigma and lack of social support leads people with AIDS to suffer more serious depression. A loving, accepting and nurturing support system is vital for people with AIDS to reach the stage of "acceptance and peace." Similarly, Ross, Tebble and Viliunas (1989) note that the lack of social support in the lives of HIV positive gay men in relationship to both their HIV status and their sexual orientation, may increase the amount of distress these men experience when compared with other terminally ill people. Their staged model of psychological reactions to HIV infection in asymptomatic homosexual men, created by synthesizing the work of Kübler-Ross (1969) and Cass (1979) on homosexual identity formation and the successful integration of a HIV positive diagnosis into the lives of gay men. The authors emphasise, as did Kübler-Ross, that their model is fluid, and the same individuals may neither experience every stage not progress beyond particular stages. Nonetheless, Minichiello (1992), following Miller and

Green (1985), objects to the application of stage models to the data collected from individuals about their reaction to a HIV positive diagnosis, calling for research that gives primacy to the distinct experiences of individuals.

In addition to Ross et al., (1989), numerous researchers argue that there are significant differences in the response of gay men to a diagnosis of HIV and people to a diagnosis of other terminal illnesses (Weitz, 1989; Turner, Hays & Coates, 1993; O'Brien, Wortman, Kessler & Joseph, 1993). These differences include the stigmatization of homosexuality and AIDS, the phenomenon of multiple loss resulting from the confinement of the epidemic to members of small connected social groups like gay men; and the uncertainty of time between diagnosis of HIV and the onset of AIDS, and the onset of AIDS and death.

Qualitative research is understood to be the most appropriate way to investigate certain type of questions. It has been characterised as being exploratory, hypothesis generating, and good at producing depth rather than breadth (Patton, 1990; Miles & Huberman, 1984). Parker and Carballo (1990) argue that a more effective approach to the issues raised by the HIV epidemic will be found in the implementation of a range of different research methods; and qualitative methods have an important role to play in answering many of the most basic questions currently confronting researchers. Discussing the nature of Australian research into AIDS, Viney and Crooks (1992) notes the "paucity of qualitative information to complement the more generalizable quantitative information."

Intimacy is defined and used in a myriad of ways in the psychological literature. It is sometimes used as an indicator of a social competence (Kurdek & Schmitt, 1987b; Brotman, 1988) or as a way of describing sexually committed relationships (e.g., Peplau & Cochran, 1981). Sometimes it is contrasted with independence as one of a pair of value orientations (Peplau, 1991), or as one side of a polarity (the other pole being isolation) in a stage theory (Erickson, 1963). Often is left undefined; seemingly being used as synonym for "close," as in "intimate emotional sharing" (e.g., Kurdek & Schmitt, 1987b; Cramer & Roach, 1988; Ahmed, 1992). Often, different definitions, understandings and uses of the term appear in the same paper (Peplau & Cochran, 1981; Kurdek & Schmitt, 1987b; Ahmed, 1992).

These definitions either lacked adequate precision or failed to capture what is commonly understood by the term. For this reason, the definition of intimacy used in this paper was taken from the work of a philosopher. Paul Gilbert (1991) says that intimacy is not created by people sharing propositional knowledge of themselves, but by sharing their "thoughts and feelings themselves." Intimate relationships are those in which people trust one another to take up an attitude of "responsive understanding" to each other's "thoughts and feelings." To understand another involves "being about to see the world in which they act as they see it."

METHOD

Research Aim

The aim of the research was to explore the types and nature of important relationships in the lives of research participants, and to discover the impact upon those relationships of participants' discovery of their HIV status. The investigative goal and the research methodology of this study arose from a formal consultative process between representatives of the National Centre for HIV Social Research and representatives of the HIV positive and gay communities.

Participants

The sample was comprised of 15 men with HIV or AIDS. All the men were residents of the cities of Brisbane or Melbourne, Australia. All the men identified themselves as exclusively homosexual. The sample was recruited through a social network system, assisted by "snowballing" techniques. An attempt was made to reach a diverse sample of men who varied in age, period of time since diagnosis, ethnic background and state of health.

The subjects' ages ranged from 23 to 45 (M = 33). Two men were diagnosed HIV positive every year from 1984 to 1992,with the exception of 1986 (0) and 1992 (1). Ten (66.7%) people identified as Anglo-Saxon Australian, two (13.3%) as Southern European, two (13.3%) as Eastern European and one (6.7%) as Aboriginal Australian. Eight (53.3%) were in full-time work, with the remainder engaged in part-time employment, receiving social benefits or some combination of the two. Thirteen (86.7%) people had at least a high school education, and thirteen (86.7%) had not had an AIDS-defining illness. All except one described himself as well at the time of the study. During the analysis, one subject died from an AIDS-related illness.

The Interview

One to one audio-taped semi-structured interviews were conducted, each taking between one and two hours. Interviews were conducted by one of the three interviewers, at a place of the participant's choosing, usually his home. All interviewers possessed formal counseling skills, several gained through counseling experience at gay men's health and AIDS organisations. Confidentiality statements were read to participants and copies signed by both the interviewer and the subject. Questions asked participants to describe the nature of their relationships with significant others, and their perception of change in those relationships since being diagnosed with HIV. Participants were specifically asked about lovers, partners, families of origins, gay families, health and support workers, but were also given an opportunity to discuss any other relationships they deemed significant. Interviewers had the discretion to use non-leading follow-up questions to further pursue particular areas of inquiry. After the completion of interviews, the researchers made note of the tone and conduct of the interview, as well as any other observations they believed would facilitate analysis of the material. Pseudonyms were assigned to all participants, and were used from the point of data analysis onward.

Data Analysis

Qualitative data obtained from the transcribed interviews was assessed through thematic content analysis. Shared meanings contained in the interviews were analyzed by grouping similar statements into content groups and abstracting the information until primary categories were defined and essential meanings emerged through the interviewing process. The relatively small amount of data collected enabled it to be hand coded. The decision to choose analytical categories from the emerging data, rather than to use predetermined categories, was made when the initial choice was made to study the issue using qualitative rather than quantitative methods. From the research team's point of view, an important advantage of qualitative research methods are their capacity to allow an understanding of problems from the participants' point of view without necessarily imposing any type of predetermined framework (Patton, 1990; Miles & Huberman, 1984). All three interviewers analyzed the data, with consensus existing amongst them regarding the identification of major themes.

RESULTS

The results show that for six men (40%) HIV catalysed a desire for clarification, enhancement and promotion of intimacy in their significant relationships. Four of the six men (66.7%) located control for bringing about desired changes in the degree of intimacy in their lives within themselves. Two men (33%) saw the means to pursue desired changes regarding the clarification, enhancement and promotion of intimacy in their lives as externally located and thus, beyond their control.

Ian, Paul, Richard, Grant, Kevin and Chris are the six men who saw HIV as a catalyst of their desire to clarify, enhance and promote intimacy in their lives. All describe difficulties in fostering and maintaining intimacy in their relationships prior to being diagnosed HIV positive.

Ian was diagnosed with HIV four months before he was interviewed. He stated that he had experienced "relationship problems for years":

> I don't trust people enough to get to know me completely, and I don't trust myself, I guess it's a self image problem, but I get very scared when people get very close. I have problems in letting people see the complete me and giving that over to someone and trusting them with it.

Letting others see him as vulnerable was difficult for Ian. Here he describes the difficulty he had accepting the allowances his employers sought to make when he experiences his first HIV related illness:

> They were trying to . . . pander to my needs, which was really lovely, but . . . I was all paranoid . . . because I wouldn't be well enough to go into work, and . . . I'd be . . . stressing about it . . . I thought they were thinking "well, what's he doing?" and each time I . . . [would] talk . . . to them about it, they in disbelief saying "Can't you see? It's ok, what do we have to do, tell us what we can do to get rid of all that stuff for you" . . . It was just me putting pressure on myself.

Paul describes a similar resistance to appearing vulnerable and accepting assistance from others prior to his diagnosis:

> I always felt I had to protect the people around me . . . that I was the one that had to be bright and . . . cheerful and everything's wonderful in life . . . to admit that there's a problem in your life is really hard . . . To open up and communicate was hard because you just weren't sure of the reaction . . . Sometimes I thought . . . I [would] get . . . people feelings sorry for me . . . or [I worried that they would] . . . not be able to cope with it . . . and I just felt that I had to up this front that everything was wonderful.

Prior to his diagnosis, Richard describes a reluctance to "ask for things" and to "be angry." He connects this difficulty with problems he had "relating to himself":

... there was a lot of anger, and I found it really hard to be angry. ...
there were other things, because relating with myself wasn't really
ever that good anyway, but I had a way of coping like people do.

He describes a distant relationship with his father, who he says

... looked[ed] more towards how I could have been to how I am, or
how I should be to how I am. I can never be exactly right for my
father. I could always be better ... I've grown up having to be very
hard on myself.

Similarly, Grant's relationship with his mother was painfully unresolved prior to his diagnosis:

I've had a very estranged relationship [with my mother] for many
years ... because when my father died when I was seven, my mother
retreated into a state of grief and showed very little emotion and
affection towards [my sister and me]. It's been an ongoing issue for
many years because she is a very cold and ungiving person ... and
that has been a source of distress and resentment and alienation to
[us] for many years ...

Kevin's mother died many years ago. His relationship with his father
had never been good:

There hasn't been much love lost between my father and myself ...
he's always chosen to pick on me, I could never do anything right in
Dad's eyes.

Kevin's disclosure of his homosexuality strained the relationship even
further:

... it was terribly difficult for a while ... but he sort of accepted my
lifestyle ... until such time as he was actually confronted with the
word "homosexual" ... [Then] I was disowned and disinherited ...
he told me in uncertain terms not to make any contact with my
family, because no one wanted to know me.

Chris's story prior to HIV bears some similarities with Kevin's. His
mother is also dead, and his father is remarried. Prior to Chris's diagnosis
with HIV, his relationship with his father was strained because of Chris's
homosexuality. Like Kevin's father, Chris's father dealt with his son's
homosexuality by not "talking about it":

They knew I was gay because I blurted that one when I was about sixteen . . . someone had sacked me and I was so depressed and I was unemployed at that stage and I just blurted out. They sent me to a psychiatrist . . . That's how they related to it . . . basically . . . that it's just a phase you are going through. [Later]

I . . . told my father that I was gay and that was that he said "I always thought" . . . They assumed that as long as you didn't talk about it . . .

For all six men, HIV catalysed a desire for clarified, enhanced and greater intimacy in their lives. Ian, Paul, Richard and Grant describe an internal locus of control for bringing about the desired change in the degree of intimacy in their lives.

Ian realized that the first step to fulfilling his desire for increased intimacy in his life acknowledging his desires and needs:

I have a friend . . . also HIV positive who . . . said: "listen, you're not approaching this in the right way. You have an overdeveloped sense of duty . . . which you have to get rid of. The time has come for you to . . . think of yourself, and your health . . . You have to be more selfish, and that's not a bad thing to develop first."

Ian's sister reacted angrily to his diagnosis with HIV. He believes that this response was due to unresolved issues she had with his homosexuality. However, he felt he couldn't "tolerate her behavior" at that time. His desire to increase the degree of intimacy in his relationship with his sister led him to "put his foot down" about seeing her in a situation in which he felt uncomfortable:

. . . I hadn't actually seen her face to face since I'd told her [about the HIV diagnosis] . . . My father was . . . arriving . . . and they wanted to get together for a family outing and I was stressing out about it because I hadn't seen either my father or my sister since telling them and . . . I just thought that I can't play the happy family bit, I need to talk about it . . . so I just put my foot down and said "look I can't do it this way. Yes, of course we can get back to that but I need something else." Which was good, because it brought it all out into the open . . . it made them realise.

Ian believes that although he still has not seen his sister, by "making [her] realize" that he was not "emotionally strong enough" at that point "to deal" with her issues, he will eventually be able to speak to re-establish close ties with her.

The shift Ian describes in his desire for intimacy in his relationship with his sister since diagnosis can also be seen in the new attitude he describes taking towards his friends:

> [HIV] changes your perception I think, in a lot of ways, and again I think a lot of good comes from it in a lot of things . . . You've got less time for triviality . . . you can set up new situations which are really good . . . I had these two friends who . . . have their problems from time to time, and I've got one in either ear, telling their sides of the story . . . and I just said "look, I can't deal with this . . . I can't afford to get stressed over it . . . " And the reaction was great, it was like: "Oh, OK."

Although he is single, Ian says that HIV has catalysed a desire to have a romantic partner. He says that he is "a lot stronger and a lot better equipped" to be in an intimate partnership than he was before his diagnosis, because HIV has given him the chance to "stop and look at [his] life," and to clear a lot of the "emotional baggage" he felt had inhibited the development of intimacy in his relationships.

Ian speculates that, rather than catalyzing his desire for increased intimacy in his life, his desire for increased intimacy may have subconsciously driven him to undertake the unsafe practices that led to his infection:

> I . . . read a book . . . [that] says that a lot of people will . . . become HIV positive to test people's love: "OK, who loves me now," and I believe this is true of myself. It's like saying "deal with this, how are you going to react." *(Is that what you wanted to do, to see if people would still be around?)* Subconsciously yeah . . . I don't know if it was the prime objective, but I think . . . to a degree that we all do that in our own way. *(And have you been reassured?)* Yeah, tenfold.

For Paul, like for Ian, the first step to increasing the amount of intimacy in his life after his diagnosis was acknowledging the vulnerability associated with being ill:

> . . . the pressure built up . . . around being this wonderful person and then I thought I'm going around the bend, I'm going to explode. That's when I went into counselling . . . [I learned] to communicate and express my feelings. . . . If someone says "Hey, let's go and do this," I say "no, I feel . . . lousy." Whereas, in the past, I would have made the effort [because I couldn't] slow down and let them know I'm not fit . . .

Being honest with others increased the intimacy in Paul's relationships as well as helped him feel better about himself:

> If you tell people and be honest with them, more often than not you get a favorable response . . . They say "OK, we'll do it another time" . . . I think it's important to be honest because you feel better about yourself . . . if you get a bad response, that's worthwhile as well because you learn from that and you can work . . . out why that person gave a bad response . . . and help them change their attitude . . .

A desire for "quality time" with his family motivated Paul to disclose to them his HIV status:

> They are your family. They will support you, they're there to help, they're going to encourage you. It's better for them to know now while you're healthy and alive, so you can have quality time with them for as long as you, y'know, may be there.

After disclosing to his family, Paul describes a period of disclosing to quite a few people because he wanted them:

> . . . to feel sorry for me . . . I wanted just to be able to say "look, I've got HIV, I'm gonna die, how do you feel about that?. . . hug me . . . feel sorry for me . . . hold me." They all showed concern, care, understanding, support . . .

Paul says that prior to HIV, he's never "had a [romantic] relationship of any length of time." However, he feels that the self development work he's undergone since diagnosis has fashioned him into "relationship material":

> In the past . . . I . . . stopped any relationship occurring . . . now I feel like, I'm in control. I've sorted out a lot of things . . . I'm ready to settle down and be intimate and love and hold someone and spend time with someone and sacrifice things in my life that I wasn't prepared to in the past . . . give them some of my space. I'm now ready to do that . . .

Richard's diagnosis "triggered off" in him a desire to "cleanse [his] inner self" and become "more open." He went overseas and, like Paul, chose to enter therapy. His experience in group and individual therapy increased his awareness of his need for self acceptance and acceptance from others:

> . . . I became more confident with myself, which of course in turn
> helped me with the virus and . . . changed my life . . . [It] opened my
> eyes to other sides of myself which would release the anger and the
> need and the love. The [therapy was] were designed to help you love
> yourself more and to help you ask for things and to help you love.

When he felt he'd become "more in touch" with himself, he returned to
Australia to disclose his HIV status to his family and to "deal" with other
unresolved family issues. Richard hopes to establish greater intimacy with
his family by working through the issues raised by his disclosure. Here he
tells of the period several weeks after disclosing his status to his family:

> I told them I wanted to talk about [HIV] . . . I [still do] . . . I've
> opened . . . up . . . doors. They have probably closed more [doors]
> than they've opened, but I keep opening them . . . *(How do they close
> doors?)* By not bringing it up until I do . . . *(How does it feel having
> to bring it up yourself all the time?)* It started off sort of like, "oh, am
> I making a big deal out of this . . . is it important?" But I feel that the
> only way I can get well is to establish better relationships with
> people, and I want to get to the point where my relationships with
> my family are comfortable for me. And they're . . . not as comfort-
> able as they could be . . . I . . . go to therapy once a week, and all my
> childhood stuff's coming up . . . and . . . I'd . . . like to talk about [it]
> with my parents . . . And by bringing up the virus I'm actually
> allowing them to bring [it] up . . . And also just to let them know that
> I'm HIV. Like "I've told you that I am, like don't just hear it as if it
> was in a dream." Because I want it to be the real thing. [I want] them
> [to] listen . . . to the fact that I'm gay too . . . that this is my life . . .
> I've never talked about myself to them. I've always found that if I've
> talked about myself it has to be something that's successful, ambi-
> tious. And I want to talk about me living with the virus, and having
> to change my life . . .

Like Ian and Paul, Richard reports that HIV catalysed a desire in him for
an intimate romantic partner. He states that he desires a relationship with
another HIV positive person in order that issues around the virus could be
understood instantly between them, leaving time for the pursuit of other
enjoyable aspects of romantic intimacy:

> I'm desperately wanting a relationship . . . But . . . they have to be
> HIV positive . . . It would be easier . . . and I . . . want the relationship
> to be . . . other things than learning about the virus . . . The virus will

be there but we can . . . explore other sides and not have to spend so much time.

Richard's words are not unlike Ian's when, after extensive discussion of his increased capacity for intimacy since diagnosis, he suggests that HIV has served its purpose in his life:

I'm getting to a point where I don't want to be HIV anymore. I am, but I don't want to be . . . I want to be like "I'm HIV positive, let's get on with it."

For Grant, diagnosis with HIV prompted a resolve to "live life to the fullest." Like Ian, Grant feels that since his diagnosis, he has little time for superficial relationships:

I feel I am no longer prepared to spend hours with people for whom I have no real rapport . . . I try to have . . . quality experiences. Which means that some friendships . . . and relationships have fallen by the wayside over the years. I would imagine this . . . would not be the case if I wasn't HIV positive.

His diagnosis also prompted Grant to seek improvement in his relationship with his mother:

. . . I felt it was important that if she wanted to have some kind of relationship with her children in her remaining years . . . that I would have to take the initiative and change things . . . And hopefully things have now been resolved. Certainly for me they have, which was very important . . . *(Has your having HIV . . . had any influence on your decision to [take the initiative]?)* Yes . . . my priorities in life [have] changed dramatically as a result of . . . AIDS.

Grant has been involved in a relationship with an HIV negative man for over a year. He says that the precautions they must take have spoiled their sexual relationship. However, while "sex and lust" were critical aspects of his romantic relationships before HIV, he finds other aspects of his current relationship compensate for the sexual difficulties:

. . . the warmth of cuddling up together at night, or the intimacy we have emotionally, the intimacy we have of just knowing each other more than compensate for the disappointments of the sexual side.

Unlike Ian, Paul, Richard and Grant, who see themselves in control of the fulfillment of their desire to clarify, enhance and promote intimacy in their lives, Kevin and Chris do not feel they are in control of the fulfillment of their intimacy desires.

Since his diagnosis, Kevin has wished for a greater degree of intimacy in his relationship with his father:

> It would be nice to have a more open relationship [with him]. I've always sort of envied the boys who have got mothers who they could relate to so well.

A close reading of Kevin's story about his father's discovery of his HIV status when Kevin was hospitalized suggests Kevin's disappointment over his father's avoidance of the issues surrounding his infection:

> . . . I told him about the HIV status, and he chose to bring up some family drama . . . that had been going on for years and I told him I didn't really have time to talk about that, . . . that I was too busy trying to sort of fight for my life . . . *(And has it been discussed since then?)* Yes, sometimes. He doesn't like to discuss it very often, but . . . I've talked about T-cells quite openly . . . and I've tried to make him . . . understand it. But I do think Dad *understands* it quite well. I think he's quite well-read on it . . . I put it to [the whole family] that . . . [having] dealt with [this illness] . . . I should have been dead by the law of averages seven years [after being infected]. Oh, they just didn't want to know about it. I promptly got told committed statistics on the number of women who die of breast cancer. There was this total barrier that came–zoomp–like a brick wall . . . I can recall Dad even changed the subject . . . [I wouldn't mind] a little more compassion that you might find from him.

Kevin repeatedly cites examples of his father's inability to "confront" Kevin's diagnosis and his related illnesses. The following excerpt is typical:

> [There's a] denial about the whole thing . . . he lost money on the stock market [and] went on about "Oh, of course I'm only trying to . . . make sure you've got money when I go." I said "I really wouldn't worry about that . . . I think I've proven that I could die before any of you" . . . This is after I'd mentioned the AIDS thing, and he just didn't want to know about it. He said "Well, that's garbage . . . what makes you think you're going to die of AIDS? . . . You want to get this out of your head." He . . . just didn't want to know about it.

Chris believes that HIV has catalyzed a desire to increase the amount of intimacy in his life:

> I need somebody. I've gone through life since the age of fourteen on my own. I just don't have anybody. I don't have commitments to anybody. . . . I have nothing, no reason to live basically . . . If I had a relationship I would have a reason to look after myself . . . I don't have any reason at the moment . . . I have not had any relationships prior to being HIV . . . I've always shied away from relationships . . . [but] I've wanted a relationship more since being [HIV].

Although HIV has catalysed a desire for increased intimacy, Chris finds it difficult to develop the qualities he believes would enable him to become intimate with others:

> It's very hard to get emotionally involved with somebody else and expect them to sort of help you . . . I don't open up to other people . . . I find it difficult to open, you know to accept help. I'll give, give, give, but I find it very difficult to receive . . . I would like to receive, yeah, but I find it difficult.

Thus, while a "very nice" man is interested in forming a relationship with him, Chris feels unable to "drop" his "protective wall" and risk getting hurt; things he knows he must do if an intimate relationship is to develop:

> I would like to get to know him more . . . [but] I find it very difficult because most of my sex is at the Saunas, anonymous one night . . . no attachment, no involvement . . . I don't get emotionally involved with anybody. Now I meet this person who wants to get involved with me, accepts me for who I am and of whom I'm fond and I'm clamming up . . . He wants to have a relationship with me, but I'm frightened of a commitment . . .

DISCUSSION

The aim of this study was to discover the types and nature of relationships of importance in the lives of gay male participants, and how these relationships were impacted upon by the participants' HIV status. The finding of this qualitative study suggest that for some of the gay men in the sample, HIV catalyses a desire to clarify, enhance and promote intimacy in their lives. The desire to clarify and promote intimacy could be seen throughout the changes the men made, or desired to make, in the types of relationships they sought with others, and the manner in which they sought to develop existing relationships. This finding is supportive of other studies which document the importance of relationships in the lives of positive gay men's lives. Further, the suggestion that one of the aspects of "emotional/social" support that positive gay men value is intimacy, and that this intimacy is valued in a wide range of important relationships, is significant. The findings also suggest that the HIV positive gay men with an inner locus of control saw self-development, often assisted by formal counseling, as a precursor to their capacity to bring about an increase in the degree of intimacy in their lives. It is possible to see this finding as confirming the existence of the fourth stage in the model of asymptomatic gay men's reactions to HIV infection described by Ross et al. (1989). Essentially, stage four posits that disclosure to significant others and the need to receive acceptance and love from them forms an essential part of resolving the crisis of an HIV positive diagnosis; a crisis which the researchers see as one on homosexual identity formation. It may be that the men in the sub-sample with an inner locus of control were interviewed during their progression through stage four of the model. Objections to stage models, as well as the vastly different time periods between diagnosis and interview that existed for the four men characterized as having an inner locus of control, however, would weigh against this interpretation. It should also be pointed out that while the model purports to describe the reactions of asymptomatic gay men, not all the men who were the subject of this paper were asymptomatic.

The focus in this paper on only six of fifteen men does not mean that intimacy was not an important issue for most of the men in the sample, but rather that HIV did not *catalyse* in these men a desire to clarify, enhance and promote intimacy in their lives. For example, Graham spent most of his interest discussing the pain of a broken relationship. He described this relationship as having been "the most important thing" in his life, and expressed interest in finding a new partner. However, Graham was not confident that HIV catalysed his desire to clarify, enhance and promote intimacy in his life:

> . . . I can't really say that . . . I'm trying to picture what it would be like not to be HIV . . . and it's been so long I can't remember what it's like . . . I think perhaps my . . . commitment to relationships has increased, perhaps because I'm HIV, but it could be just that I'm ten

years older . . . Maybe I've just matured, rather than the HIV has changed it.

Two cautions must be issued with regard to the findings. The small sample size means it is not warranted to apply the findings to the population of HIV positive gay men. The importance of the findings lies in their capacity to suggest areas for further quantitative exploration, as well as their capacity to add depth to existing quantitative studies. In addition, doubt remains regarding the HIV as catalyst thesis because of the suggestion made in Ian and Richard's interviews that HIV gave them the opportunity, or the excuse, to act out their desires for intimacy, rather than the virus catalysing those desires. Research designed to investigate the validity of the HIV as catalyst thesis, as well as this alternative construction, would be welcomed.

REFERENCES

Acevedo, J.R. (1986) Impact of risk reduction on mental health. In L. McKusick (ed). *What to do about AIDS.* Berkeley, CA: University of California Press, pp. 95-102.

Berger, R.M. (1990) Men Together: Understanding the Gay Couple. *Journal of Homosexuality, 19(3),* 31-49.

Blumstein, P. & Schwartz, P. (1983) *American Couples.* New York: William Morrow.

Blyth, B.J (1983) Social support networks in health care and health promotion. In J.K. Whittaker & J. Garabarino (eds), *Social support networks,* New York: Aldine, pp. 107-133.

Brotman, A. & Forstein, M. (1988) AIDS Obsession in Depressed Homosexuals. *Psychosomatics, 29(4),* 428-431.

Cass, V.C. (1979) Homosexual identity formation: A theoretical model. *Journal of Homosexuality, 4,* 219-235.

Cramer, D.W. & Roach, A.J. (1988) Coming Out to Mom and Dad: A Study of Gay Males and Their Relationships with Their Parents. *Journal of Homosexuality, 15(3/4),* 79-91.

D'Augelli, A. (1983) Social support networks in mental health. In J.K. Whittaker & J. Garabarino (eds), *Social support networks,* New York: Aldine, pp. 73-106.

Dannecker, M. (1981) *Theories of Homosexuality.* London: Gay Men's Press.

Erikson, E. (1963) *Childhood and Society.* New York: Norton.

Gilbert, P. (1991) *Human Relationships.* Oxford: Basis Blackwell.

Gonsiorek, J.C. & Rudolph, J.R. (1991) Homosexuality Identity: Coming Out and Other Developmental Events. In J.C. Gonsiorek & J.D. Weinrich (eds.), *Homosexuality: Research Implications for Public Policy,* Newbury Park, California: Sage Publications, pp. 161-176.

Gottlieb, B.H. (1983) Social support as a focus for integrative research in psychology. *American Psychologist, 38*, 278-287.

Hammersmith, S. & Weinberg, M. (1973) Homosexual identity: Commitment, adjustment and significant others. *Sociometry, 36*, 56-79.

Jacobs, J.A. & Tedford, W.H. (1980) Factors affecting self-esteem of the homosexual individual. *Journal of Homosexuality, 5*, 373-382.

Kübler-Ross, E. (1969) *On death and dying.* London: Tavistock.

Kübler-Ross, E. (1987) *AIDS–The ultimate challenge.* New York: Macmillan.

Kurdek, L.A. & Schmitt, J.P. (1987b) Perceived emotional support from family and friends in members of homosexual, married and heterosexual cohabiting couples. *Journal of Homosexuality, 14(3/4)*, pp. 57-68.

Mattison, A.M. & McWhirter, D.P. (1990) Emotional Impact of AIDS: Male Couples and Their Families. In B. Voeller, J.M. Reinisch & M. Gottlieb (eds.) *AIDS and Sex: An Integrated Biomedical and Biobehavioural Approach.* The Kinsey Institute Series, J.M. Reinisch General Editor. Vol. IV. New York, Oxford: Oxford University Press.

McWhirter, D.P. & Mattison, A.M. (1984) *The Male Couple: How Relationships Develop.* Englewood Cliffs, NJ: Prentice-Hall.

Miles, M.B. & Huberman, M.A. (1984) *Qualitative data analysis: A source book of new methods.* Beverly Hills, California: Sage.

Miller, D. & Green, J. (1985) Psychological support and counselling for patients with AIDS. *Genitourinary Medicine, 61*, 273-278.

Minichiello, V. (1992) Gay Men Discuss Social Issues and Personal Concerns. In E. Timewell, V. Minichiello & D. Plummer (eds), *AIDS in Australia.* Australia: Prentice Hall, pp. 142-161.

Namir, S., Wolcott, D.L., Fawzy, F. & Alumbaugh, M. (1987) Coping with AIDS: Psychological and Health Implications. *Journal of Applied Social Psychology, 17*, 309-328.

Nicholson, W.D. & Long, B.C. (1990) Self-Esteem, Social Support, Internalized Homophobia, and Coping Strategies of HIV+ Gay Men. *Journal of Consulting and Clinical Psychology, 58(6)*, 873-876.

O'Brien, K., Wortmen, C.B., Kessler, R.C. & Joseph, J.G. (1993) Social Relationships of Men at Risk for AIDS. *Social Science Medicine, 36(9)*, 1161-1167.

Parker, R.G. & Carballo, M. (1990) Qualitative Research on Homosexual and Bisexual Behaviour Relevant to HIV/AIDS. *The Journal of Sex Research, 27(4)*, 497-525.

Patton, M.Q. (1990) *Qualitative Evaluation and Research Methodology.* Newbury Park, California: Sage Publications.

Peplau, L.A. (1991) Lesbian and Gay Relationships. In J.C. Gonsiorek & J.D. Weinrich (eds.), *Homosexuality: Research Implications for Public Policy.* Newbury Park, California: Sage Publications, pp. 177-196.

Peplau, L.A. & Cochran, S.D. (1981) Value Orientations in the Intimate Relations of Gay Men. *Journal of Homosexuality, 6(3)*, 1-19.

Ross, M.W. (1990) The relationships between life events and mental health in homosexual men. *Journal of Clinical Psychology, 46*, 402-411.

Ross, M., Tebble, W. & Viliunas, D. (1989) Staging of Psychological Reactions to HIV Infections in Asymptomatic Homosexual Men. *Journal of Psychology & Human Sexuality, 2(1)*, 93-104.

Schaeffer, S. & Coleman, E. (1992) Shifts in Meaning, Purpose and Values Following a Diagnosis of Human Immunodeficiency Virus (HIV) Infection Among Gay Men. *Journal of Psychology & Human Sexuality, 5(1/2)*, 13-29.

Schmitt, J.P. & Kurdek, L.A. (1987a) Personality Correlates of Positive Identity and Relationships Involvement in Gay Men. *Journal of Homosexuality, 13(4)*, pp. 101-109.

Teguis, A. & Ahmed, P. (1992) Living with AIDS. In P. Ahmed (ed.) *Living and Dying with AIDS*. New York, London: Plenum Press, pp. 3-18.

Turner, H.A., Hays, R.B. & Coates, T.J. (1993) Determinants of Social Support Among Gay Men: The Context of AIDS. *Journal of Health and Social Behavior, 34*, 37-53.

Viney, L. & Crooks, L. (1992) The Psychological Meaning. In E. Timewell, V. Minichiello & D. Plummer (eds.) *AIDS in Australia*. Australia: Prentice Hall, pp. 108-124.

Weinberg, M.S. & Williams, C.J. (1974) *Male Homosexuals: Their Problems and Adaptations*. New York: Oxford University Press.

Weitz, R. (1989) Uncertainty and the Lives of Persons with AIDS. *Journal of Health and Social Behaviour, 30*, 270-281.

Wolcott, D.L., Namir, S., Fawzy, F.I., Gottelieb, M.S. & Mitsuyasu, R.T. (1986) Illness concerns, attitudes towards homosexuality, and social support in gay men with AIDS. *General Hospital Psychiatry, 8*, 395-403.

Zich, J. & Temoshok, L. (1987) Perceptions of social support in men with AIDS and ARC: Relationships with distress and hardiness. *Journal of Applied Social Psychology, 17*, 193-215.

Issues of Isolation and Intimacy for the HIV Infected, Sexually Addicted Gay Male in Group Psychotherapy

Michele M. Fontaine, MA

SUMMARY. The pertinent issues of isolation and intimacy with sexually addicted, HIV infected gay males was researched from the perspective of group psychotherapy as a treatment modality. The purpose of the article was to highlight shame based feelings associated with being sexually addicted and HIV diagnosed with the subsequent behaviors of isolation and difficulties with intimacy. The group model is examined as a means towards alleviating isolation and helping the client form new ways towards bonding and forming intimacy. Group interventions are seen to be helpful in lessening sexual compulsivity, creating new forms of relating and providing a safe environment for an individual dealing with HIV disease. *[Single or multiple copies of this article are available from The Haworth Document Delivery Service: 1-800-342-9678, 9:00 a.m. - 5:00 p.m. (EST).]*

Isolation and intimacy in the field of addiction have been examined and explored from various angles. When adding the specific issues of sexual addiction, a HIV diagnosis and homosexuality, these two issues take on a new perspective. Group psychotherapy has had positive results in treating

Michele M. Fontaine is affiliated with Greenwich House, AIDS Mental Health Project, New York, NY.

[Haworth co-indexing entry note]: "Issues of Isolation and Intimacy for the HIV Infected, Sexually Addicted Gay Male in Group Psychotherapy." Fontaine, Michele M. Co-published simultaneously in *Journal of Psychology & Human Sexuality* (The Haworth Press, Inc.) Vol. 7, No. 1/2, 1995, pp. 181-190; and: *HIV/AIDS and Sexuality* (ed: Michael W. Ross) The Haworth Press, Inc., 1995, pp. 181-190; and: *HIV/AIDS and Sexuality* (ed: Michael W. Ross) Harrington Park Press, an imprint of The Haworth Press, Inc., 1995, pp. 181-190. *[Single or multiple copies of this article are available from The Haworth Document Delivery Service: 1-800-342-9678, 9:00 a.m. - 5:00 p.m. (EST).]*

181

addiction, sexual dysfunctions and in alleviating isolation from whatever origin. For the HIV infected, gay male battling with mortality concerns, sexual orientation and a sexual addiction, group psychotherapy can be distinctly helpful. The inevitable isolation that comes from these issues can be lessened through group psychotherapy helping the client develop new ways of relating and eventually finding some means towards intimacy.

LITERATURE

Quadland (1985) has defined sexual compulsivity as a lack of control over one's sexual behavior. Love and affection are often confused with sexual behaviors and the compulsivity is fueled, so to speak, by anxieties based on loneliness and fears of intimacy. A history of long term relationships is nonexistent and chemical abuse is often involved in the client's behavior thus compounding the problem of the sexual compulsivity (Quadland, 1985). Intimacy created in a group situation, as Quadland stipulates (1985), helps to reduce the inhibitions in forming relationships, reduces isolation, confronts resistance and encourages new behaviors.

In reviewing the literature, sexual compulsivity, paraphilia and sexual addiction often overlap each other. According to Levine, Risen and Althof (1990) paraphilia is a disorder of intention. It represents an impairment in the bonding function, courtship disorders and is considered an erotic form of hatred based on childhood trauma. Sexual compulsivity falls under the third criterion of paraphilia. Levine et al. (1990) define sexual compulsivity as manifesting around the arousal point and in the hunting aspect of the behavior. Sexual compulsivity is viewed as a paraphilia due to the aggression component Levine et al. (1990) refer to in their overall definition.

Pincu (1989) looks at sexual dysfunction using an addictive model. Anxiety reduction is alleviated as with any addiction through all six phases in addiction: the fix, excitement, increase in tolerance, withdrawal and loss of control followed by denial. Anxiety is sexualized and intimacy and intensity are confused. A behaviorally oriented group approach is recommended so as to reduce the client's pain (Pincu, 1989).

Chemical abuse and sexual compulsivity are often correlated in the literature. Stall, McKusick, Wiley, Coates and Ostrow (1986) researched four areas in regards to alcohol, drug use and safe sex practices. Chemical abuse and sexual activity were examined from the perspectives of four constructs: disinhibition, aphrodisiac qualities, personality traits and a social context. The ritual behavior under the area of social context was particularly similar to the acting out behavior of the sexually compulsive client. Alcohol and drug abuse were also seen to have a significant role in unsafe sexual practices (Stall et al., 1986).

Research conducted over the correlation between sexuality and death and/or HIV has increased with the advent of the AIDS epidemic. Quadland and Shattls (1987) theoretically researched sexual control, sexuality and AIDS and noted this association. Sexual compulsivity was seen to express an inner need over and above a genital urge. An example of an inner need was alleviation of anxiety created by a HIV diagnosis. The sexual activity was seen to increase the loneliness of the clients thus creating more of a need to eliminate this pain through sexual acting out. The group psychotherapy approach that Quadland and Shattls (1987) used helped to lower the frequency of the sexual compulsivity and to manage sex in a life-enhancing way.

Kelly et al. (1991) have also examined the relationship between a HIV diagnosis and sexual behavior. Two types of behaviors were looked at in relation to these issues: avoidance with a fighting spirit and an anxious preoccupation/sense of helplessness. The latter behavior was seen as correlating with a poorer psychological state and much more closely linked with the HIV infected group examined. Higher rates of at risk sexual behavior were also noted from this specific clientele.

Shame based, sexual behaviors have been examined in great depth from an addictive perspective by Carnes (1985). Post traumatic stress syndrome associated with childhood abuse can cause displaced anxiety. A HIV diagnosis can also create post traumatic stress syndrome. A fusion of sex with emotions around nurturance, fear, loneliness and vulnerability is the result. These are very similar emotions seen in an individual with a HIV diagnosis suffering from post traumatic stress syndrome.

Conflict avoidance is constantly at play and with a sex addict, this manifests through compulsive behavior. According to Carnes (1985) sex can make isolation bearable. The sexual addict is often hypercritical and judgmental showing no acceptance for personal responsibility. The sexual addiction is comprised of preoccupation, ritualization, compulsive sexual behavior and despair. Carnes (1985) believes that the sex addict must develop roots in a caring community so as to lessen the isolation and learn new ways to relate in a non-sexual manner.

Coming to terms with one's sexual orientation, such as with a gay person, compounds the sexual issues even further due to the never ending problems of shame and acceptance. Anger and shame are an integral piece of the sexual addiction which is constantly masked by the excitement, arousal and trance of the acting out episode (Carnes, 1985).

Abandonment for this population is the very basis of sexual addiction. Intimacy is often perceived as the potential loss of reality and integrity. Carnes (1985) proposes four core beliefs for the sex addict: the client views him/herself as a bad person; they see themselves as unlovable;

needs will never be met if dependent on someone else; sex is the only important need.

Schaef (1989) posits similar ideas on the subject of sexual addiction. She views the problem from a more societal point of view and she feels that our repressed, homophobic culture contributes to more sexual compulsivity. Society is equally repressed and diseased in some way with sexual addiction forming an integral part of the fabric of this culture. In thinking about society's reaction to the AIDS epidemic and to homosexuality, her position is fairly clear. More shame is associated with sex addiction compared to chemical or other addiction yet it is almost promoted and validated in our culture. The family contributes to the disease and the breaking of the family's denial is critical (Schaef, 1989). Schaef (1989) and Carnes (1985) both believe in approaching sexual addiction from a family systems' approach.

Schaffer and Zimmerman (1990) speak of the flawed self-belief system of the sex addict–a similar position to Carnes (1985). The shattered sense of self that Schaffer and Zimmerman (1990) refer to when the client receives their HIV diagnosis is further enhanced by the sexual addiction. The alleviation of pain from the intense isolation of sexual addiction and being HIV infected is paramount and is undertaken via ritualization, sexual preoccupation, compulsive sexual behavior and resulting despair– the same patterns discussed by Carnes (1985). The use of group therapy to reinforce positive coping skills before the dysfunctional sexual behavior is launched, is a large part of Schaffer and Zimmerman's (1990) theory.

BASIC THEMES

In 1991 at an outpatient psychotherapy clinic in New York City it became clear that in addition to the chemical abuse and HIV related issues being treated, sexual behaviors were becoming more prominent in the clinical material. Increased sexual compulsivity associated with the HIV diagnosis and subsequent anxiety, shame and isolation were being brought up more frequently. Significant ramifications for safe sex practices, transmission and reinfection to the client were being presented. A psychotherapy group was proposed and initiated in February, 1992.

To date, there have been over sixty sessions. The group was originally facilitated by two facilitators, one male with a Master's in Psychology and one female with a Master's in Counseling. After approximately four months of sessions, the male facilitator resigned from the agency and the female facilitator has remained as the only facilitator. The group was able to make this transition smoothly while issues of abandonment surfaced quite readily with the male facilitator's exit. Three of the six members are the core or original members. Members who left the group did so because of drug relapses and escalated sexual acting out behavior, poor attendance with subsequent discharge from the clinic or because of death. Every member currently, with the exception of one, has had a substance abuse history with one of the six still actively abusing alcohol. Three of the six members have reported sexual abuse as children while one of the remaining three has been witness to both sexual and physical abuse in the family. Themes that have emerged and continue to present themselves involve the shame and anxiety of being HIV infected, gay and sexually compulsive with subsequent isolation; inability to form intimate relationships; poor boundaries; loneliness; self-image distortion; death and dying; HIV disclosure and homophobia.

GROUP ISSUES AND THEORY

Bennis and Shepard (1956) formulated a group theory that has been applicable over the years to many groups and specifically to the group in question. They have divided the group process into various phases as listed sequentially: dependence-submission, counterdependence, resolution, enchantment, disenchantment and consensual validation. The dependence-submission phase is marked by content focused on external issues and rule setting. The counterdependence phase starts to show distrust of the facilitator and a group search for a consensus mechanism. The resolution phase displays pairing among members and the development of an internal authority. The enchantment phase shows more pairing but also flight responses and a high degree of suggestibility. The disenchantment phase is marked by levels of high anxiety, intimacy requirements/needs and the restructuring of the group into two distinct camps primarily made up of the personals and the counterpersonals. The consensual validation phase shows signs of acceptance and understanding for all involved and a diminishing of ties based on personal orientation or needs.

The group has moved in a circular way, not a linear way (typical of most group process) throughout these phases during the sixty or more sessions of its existence. The members have gone through these phases with a striking rapidity due to their sense of urgency over time, deterioration and dying from their HIV illness as well as their similar compulsive personality structures.

Intimacy has been flirted with and pairing has resulted as would be seen in the phase of enchantment. On the other hand, intimacy has been avoided throughout the life of the group with open displays of a need for control, power and impeachment of the facilitator, as seen in the resolution phase. Abandonment issues have been strikingly consistent and present. Members have become more noticeably ill from HIV disease causing periodic absence. On the other hand absences and lateness are also attributed to fears of increasing intimacy and fears of dying. Abandonment fears would be correlated to increased absenteeism and flight and would fall into the disenchantment phase.

The significant lack of contact of a non-sexual nature for these members with other men has come up frequently in the process. Long term relations have often failed, not lasting beyond three to four months. Impairment in bonding and forming intimacy overall have been a running theme and have gotten played out in the dependence-submission phase, an earlier phase, where external material is preferred over internal material and/or more intimacy among members.

The use of ritualization in descriptions of the sexual acting out process has been consistent throughout the sessions but less so as compulsive sexual behavior overall has been lessened. As members have become more consciously aware of their ritualized and often dissociative behaviors, their sexual acting out has lost its appeal and has significantly lessened.

The patterns of being and feeling helpless in the face of the individual member's sexual problems and being HIV infected has predominated over a more fighting stance. The usual behaviors of fight-flight as seen in the disenchantment phase are more stressed on the flight response with this group due to the overriding feelings of helplessness and inability to tolerate minimal levels of anxiety.

Denial levels over mortality concerns have run high from the start of group to the present. A need to project an almost false integrity, particularly with one member who happens to be the most educated and from the highest socio-economic class in the group, has been a constant behavior. As a result of this he has insulated and isolated himself further from the potential intimacy with other members. This particular member seems to be perpetually locked in the resolution phase where exiting the facilitator is a primary concern so as to gain more control in the group. Tremendous fear around his HIV status as well as shame about his sexual practices have helped to augment this projective pattern. A need to maintain some form of control overall is paramount for this member typical of the resolution phase.

The resolution phase also exhibits a need to define the facilitator's role and the group's identity. This is often repeated with this group so as to avoid the more pertinent group task of bonding and intimacy and breaking down denial over mortality fears. Overall, complete trust and dependence on others for meeting needs is still a long ways off even after sixty sessions.

The disenchantment phase has manifested via classic behaviors of fight-flight particularly around mortality areas. More anxiety reactions have also manifested in the group as some intimacy potential between members has just started to surface. This material has only recently been evident for the past two to three months of the total seventeen months of the group's existence. The perceived threat to self-esteem that more group involvement implies in this phase is especially poignant for someone sexually addicted who is already terrified of engulfment, too much bonding and loss of self.

Consensual validation has been touched on by the members only recently (session number fifty to the present). Members are now attempting to start to bond and to reflect back to each other more conscious awareness of each other. Sexual behavior is being discussed more frankly by most members. HIV concerns are still in a shroud of denial yet as individual members become more apparently ill the denial is dissipated and discussion follows despite the painfulness of it and the high levels of anxiety that ensue.

CONCLUSION

The use of group psychotherapy as a treatment modality for the HIV infected, sexually addicted gay male is one of the most viable interventions for this special population. The common themes of shame and isolation in the group in question are addressed in Quadland's article (1985). Fears of intimacy abound for the client who has great difficulty forming relationships, bonding with others, particularly of the same sex. An impairment of bonding as described by Levine et al. (1990) has been a major issue in this group.

For an individual who is HIV diagnosed, self-image concerns are in the forefront. As with most of the clients in this particular group, a substance abuse history has been part of the clients' history. One member is still actively abusing alcohol. Stall et al. (1986), Quadland (1985) and Carnes (1985) speak about the correlation between sexual compulsivity, unsafe sex and chemical abuse. Many of the recovered clients in the group have been able to see how they have substituted their chemical abuse for sexual addiction or sexual compulsivity. The one active client has connected the two behaviors as inseparable in that he cannot act out sexually until he is intoxicated from alcohol.

The helplessness that Kelly et al. (1991) refer to with the sexual addict is amplified with the threat of increased physical deterioration from HIV disease. In this group's form of helplessness, sexual compulsivity has increased. Loneliness, which both Carnes (1985) and Schaef (1989) refer to with an individual who is sexually addicted, is also exaggerated for a client who is alone, HIV infected and gay. In coming into a group situation where tremendous opportunity is available for identification and support, the client's homophobia, sense of unworthiness from both the sex addiction and the HIV diagnosis can be alleviated. Members in the group in question have bonded with each other outside of the group and found ways to lessen anxiety levels from helplessness instead of using sex and/or chemicals.

Anxiety reduction according to Pincu (1989) is the primary goal for the sexually addicted client. A group setting can increase anxiety levels at times yet does so in a protective environment. In this environment the client can gain necessary detachment from the trance-like behavior of the sexual addiction, see the behavior as failing to eliminate shameful feelings and feelings of isolation and attempt new ways of lessening the anxiety. As stated previously, sexual compulsivity is beyond a genital urge and group psychotherapy can help the client to find new ways of forming intimacy and to manage sex in a more life enhancing way (Quadland and Shattls, 1987).

The post traumatic stress disorder resulting from child abuse has been at play in the group. Most of the clients have experienced some form of abuse and could be categorized as suffering post traumatic stress disorder as outlined in the *DSM-III-R*. A HIV diagnosis can also cause similar symptoms. According to Carnes (1985), this disorder for the sex addict can create a fusion of sex with feelings of nurturance, fear, loneliness and vulnerability. The need for the client to be in a caring community is critical especially if the client is suffering from a two pronged form of post traumatic stress disorder such as the membership in this group. Group therapy can provide that community and has proven successful in helping the clients to separate out sex and all the other feelings associated with the disorder, primarily loneliness and fear.

The shattered sense of self referred to by Schaffer and Zimmerman (1990) seen in the sexually compulsive individual who is also dealing with a HIV diagnosis and increasing mortality awareness, has been demonstrated in the group repeatedly. Once more the group setting has helped to create a caring environment that is safe with constant identification breaking down denial and subsequent isolation.

In the time span from 1985-1991 little has been written regarding the sexually addicted/compulsive, HIV infected gay male. In the literature presented some common themes have emerged: loneliness or isolation, difficulties with intimacy, shame and feelings of unworthiness. Groups in the past, with less challenging populations, have helped to put together an environment where clients have been able to allow specific anxieties to surface, examine these anxieties and experiment at ways to alleviate them in a much healthier fashion. In this particular group, new rituals have been designed via the group process itself helping the clients to dissipate and lessen the potency of their long term, sexually addictive rituals. Group structuring through rule setting and by the group structure in and of itself has also helped to provide such a shame based and isolated client with a safe, protective and predictable environment. This point alone, in its simplicity, has probably been the single and most important part of the therapeutic process.

Sexual compulsivity as defined from the perspective of this clientele and the group described is seen as an addictive response similar to a chemical addiction involving deeply rooted belief systems and early developmental stages. Treatment needs to expose these distorted belief systems in a caring and safe environment. This provides an arena for the client to start to experiment at forming new, healthier belief systems and change dysfunctional behaviors.

Intimacy issues have been a large part of the group process for a long time. For the sexually compulsive/addicted client whose intimacy issues are skewed and distorted, group intervention has proven to be effective. The new and specialized population of the HIV infected, sexually addicted gay male has also benefitted from group intervention. This type of client will continue to do so as new forms of intimacy are explored. Isolation from the client's sexual addiction and HIV diagnosis is diffused and eventually alleviated by virtue of the group setting.

REFERENCES

Bennis, W. G. & Shepard, H. A. (1956). A Theory of Group Development. *Human Relations, 9*, 415-437.

Carnes, P. (1985). *Out of the Shadows: Understanding Sexual Addiction.* Minneapolis: CompCare Publishers.

Kelly, B., Dunne, M., Raphael, B., Buckman, C., Zoucrazi, S., Smith, S., & Statham, D. (1991). Relationships Between Mental Adjustment to HIV Diagnosis, Psychological Morbidity and Sexual Behaviour. *British Journal of Clinical Psychology, 30*(4), 370-371.

Levine, S. B., Risen, C. B., & Althof, S. E. (1990). Essay on the Diagnosis and Nature of Paraphilia. *Journal of Sex and Marital Therapy, 16*(2), 89-102.

Pincu, L. (1989). Sexual Compulsivity in Gay Men: Controversy and Treatment. *Journal of Counseling and Development, 68*(1), 63-66.

Quadland, M. C. (1985). *Compulsive Sexual Behavior: Definition of a Problem and an Approach to Treatment, 11*(2), 121-132.

Quadland, M. C., & Shattls, W. D. (1987). *AIDS, Sexuality and Sexual Control, 14*(1-2), 277-298.

Schaef, A. W. (1989). *Escape from Intimacy.* San Francisco: Harper.

Schaffer, S. D., & Zimmerman, M. L. (1990). *The Sexual Addict: A Challenge for the Primary Care Provider, 15*(6), 25-33.

Stall, R., McKusick, L., Wiley, J., Coates, T., & Ostrow, D. (1986). *Alcohol and Drug Use During Sexual Activity and Compliance with Safe Sex Guidelines for AIDS: The AIDS Behavioral Project, 13*(4), 357-371.

Index

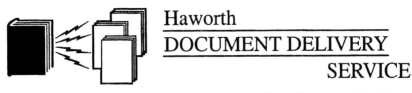

Haworth
DOCUMENT DELIVERY
SERVICE

This new service provides a single-article order form for any article from a Haworth journal.

- *Time Saving:* No running around from library to library to find a specific article.
- *Cost Effective:* All costs are kept down to a minimum.
- *Fast Delivery:* Choose from several options, including same-day FAX.
- *No Copyright Hassles:* You will be supplied by the original publisher.
- *Easy Payment:* Choose from several easy payment methods.

Open Accounts Welcome for . . .
- Library Interlibrary Loan Departments
- Library Network/Consortia Wishing to Provide Single-Article Services
- Indexing/Abstracting Services with Single Article Provision Services
- Document Provision Brokers and Freelance Information Service Providers

---

MAIL or *FAX* THIS ENTIRE ORDER FORM TO:

Haworth Document Delivery Service
The Haworth Press, Inc.
10 Alice Street
Binghamton, NY 13904-1580

or **FAX:** (607) 722-6362
or **CALL:** 1-800-3-HAWORTH
(1-800-342-9678; 9am-5pm EST)

PLEASE SEND ME PHOTOCOPIES OF THE FOLLOWING SINGLE ARTICLES:

1) Journal Title: _____
    Vol/Issue/Year: _____ Starting & Ending Pages: _____
Article Title: _____
_____

2) Journal Title: _____
    Vol/Issue/Year: _____ Starting & Ending Pages: _____
Article Title: _____
_____

3) Journal Title: _____
    Vol/Issue/Year: _____ Starting & Ending Pages: _____
Article Title: _____
_____

4) Journal Title: _____
    Vol/Issue/Year: _____ Starting & Ending Pages: _____
Article Title: _____
_____

(See other side for Costs and Payment Information)

COSTS: Please figure your cost to order quality copies of an article.

1. Set-up charge per article: $8.00
   ($8.00 × number of separate articles) _____

2. Photocopying charge for each article:

   1-10 pages: $1.00 _____

   11-19 pages: $3.00 _____

   20-29 pages: $5.00 _____

   30+ pages: $2.00/10 pages _____

3. Flexicover (optional): $2.00/article _____

4. Postage & Handling: US: $1.00 for the first article/
   $.50 each additional article _____

   Federal Express: $25.00 _____

   Outside US: $2.00 for first article/
   $.50 each additional article _____

5. Same-day FAX service: $.35 per page _____

   GRAND TOTAL: _____

METHOD OF PAYMENT: (please check one)

❏ Check enclosed   ❏ Please ship and bill. PO # _____
   (sorry we can ship and bill to bookstores only! All others must pre-pay)

❏ Charge to my credit card: ❏ Visa; ❏ MasterCard; ❏ American Express;

Account Number: _____   Expiration date: _____

Signature: X _____

Name: _____   Institution: _____

Address: _____

_____

City: _____   State: _____   Zip: _____

Phone Number: _____   FAX Number: _____

MAIL or *FAX* THIS ENTIRE ORDER FORM TO:

Haworth Document Delivery Service	**or FAX:** (607) 722-6362
The Haworth Press, Inc.	**or CALL:** 1-800-3-HAWORTH
10 Alice Street	(1-800-342-9678; 9am-5pm EST)
Binghamton, NY 13904-1580	